This book should be returned to any branch of the
Lancashire County Library on or before the date

- 9 MAR 2020

1 7 AUG 2016

- 1 JUL 2017

13 SEP 2017

2 9 DEC 2017

- 4 FEB 2019

1 2 APR 2019

1 5 MAY 2019

t
fr

'A
hist

tions that arise as she digs into   *Times*

LAN

D0177368

3011813095225 6

'Montross explores the practical, emotional, and philosophical challenges of working with patients whose illnesses of the mind are often intractable.' **The New Yorker**

'These stories are fascinating in the macabre way that psychiatric case studies can be, but *Falling into the Fire* is not a mere catalogue of human oddities... Her patients' neurons are certainly misfiring, but these individuals have just as certainly led beleaguered lives with fractured relationships... Powerful.' **Washington Post**

'*Falling into the Fire* is as good an account of the labyrinth of mental health care as you're likely to read. Montross writes beautifully about the deep-seated illnesses that challenge therapist and psychiatrists.' **Daily Beast**

'[Montross's] intriguing analysis is anchored by [a] humble and empathetic voice.' **Publishers Weekly**

'Poetic... This beautifully written book doesn't offer answers but rather encourages compassion.' **Library Journal**

'Montross writes with a dramatic flair, ever empathetic.' **Kirkus Reviews**

FALLING

INTO THE

FIRE

{ A PSYCHIATRIST'S ENCOUNTERS
WITH THE MIND IN CRISIS }

CHRISTINE MONTROSS

ONEWORLD

A ONEWORLD BOOK

First published in Great Britain and the Commonwealth by Oneworld Publications, 2014
This edition published by Oneworld Publications in 2015

First published in the United States and Canada by Penguin Press,
a member of the Penguin Group (USA) Inc.

Paperback ISBN: 978-1-78074-641-8
Ebook ISBN: 978-1-78074-367-7

Interior design by Nicole LaRoche
Printed and bound in Great Britain by Clays Ltd, St Ives plc

Oneworld Publications
10 Bloomsbury Street, London WC1B 3SR

The names of all patients and certain details of their stories have been changed in order to preserve confidentiality. For the same reason, the names of some of my colleagues have also been changed.

For Deborah and my children,
who multiply my life's joy

And for my patients,
who help me to never take that joy for granted

To acknowledge the reality of affliction means saying to oneself: '. . . There is nothing that I might not lose. It could happen at any moment that what I am might be abolished and be replaced by anything whatsoever of the filthiest and most contemptible sort.' To be aware of this in the depths of one's soul is to experience non-being. It is the state of extreme and total humiliation which is also the condition for passing over into truth.

– Simone Weil

They called me mad, and I called them mad, and damn them, they outvoted me.

– The Restoration playwright Nathaniel Lee,
regarding his committal to Bethlem Royal Hospital

[CONTENTS]

PROLOGUE
Bedlam   1

CHAPTER ONE
The Woman Who Needed a Zipper   19

CHAPTER TWO
Fifty-Thousand-Dollar Skin   67

CHAPTER THREE
Your Drugs Take Away the Love   97

CHAPTER FOUR
I've Hidden All the Knives   135

CHAPTER FIVE
Dancing Plagues and Double Impostors   163

EPILOGUE
Into the Fire, Into the Water   207

ACKNOWLEDGMENTS   217
BIBLIOGRAPHY   221
INDEX   227

FALLING INTO THE FIRE

Bedlam

Canst thou not minister to a mind diseased?
— Shakespeare, *Macbeth*

I n early January, Charles Harold Wrigley, a twenty-two-year-old gas engineer, was brought by his family to the psychiatric hospital. 'The patient is extremely depressed', the evaluating physician wrote. 'He sat with his hand on his forehead as if in pain during my interview. He says everything he does is wrong and that he is very miserable.' A second doctor's note adds, 'I am informed . . . that the patient has suicidal tendencies and since he has been [at] this hospital has attempted to strangle himself.' Notes like these are familiar to me. As a psychiatrist, I have seen countless patients in emergency rooms, inpatient units, and outpatient offices whom I might have described in nearly identical terms. This patient's symptoms are not striking; however, the familiarity of the description is, considering that Charles Harold Wrigley was evaluated and treated at England's Bethlem Royal Hospital in 1890.

Before I became a doctor, I had more faith in medicine. I thought that medical school and residency would teach me the body's intricacies, its capacities to heal and to falter, and all of our various methods of intervening. Once I mastered these, I thought, I would really *know* something. That has turned out to be partially true. I know many more things about the body – its wonders and its failings – than I could ever have imagined. But as a doctor, I have emerged from my training with a shaken faith. If I hold my trust in medicine up to the light, I see that it is full of cracks and seams. In some places it is luminous. In others it is opaque. And yet I practice.

At times this doubt is disillusioning. More often, however, I've come to view the questions that arise as a vital component of the work of medicine. My faith in medical knowledge has shifted into a faith that the effort – the *practice* – of medicine is worthwhile. I cannot always say with certainty whether the course of treatment I prescribe will heal; I cannot always locate with precision the source of my patients' symptoms and suffering. Still, I believe that trying – to heal my patients and to dwell amid the many questions that their illnesses generate – is a worthwhile pursuit.

I have found that one of the gifts of medicine is that it allows those who practice it to participate in the purest and most vulnerable moments of human life. As doctors we share in the utter joy of birth, the irrepressible relief of a normal scan or a benign biopsy. We deliver earth-shattering diagnoses. We accompany people to their deaths. In these moments there is not much room for the protective or insulating layers that people – all of us – put upon ourselves in our daily lives. Joy is joy, and grief is grief, and fear is fear; and in the context of medicine, those emotions are often at their most primitive and raw. As an inpatient psychiatrist, I treat people who are in moments of profound crisis. The majority of them are hospitalized because they might not be safe otherwise. I do not lose sight of the fact that my patients come to me in these precarious states.

I am a few years into my psychiatric practice. Relatively speaking, I am new to the job. Every day that I go to work on the inpatient psychiatry wards, I encounter people who are despondent, or terrified, or raving mad. I see people whose lives have been ruined by addiction. I hear unfathomable things that people have done to others, from familial betrayals to brutal attacks. I talk with people who, more than they have ever wanted anything, want to die. It is not a dull job.

This book was written over the course of my residency in psychiatry and in my first years as an attending psychiatrist. As a house officer, I worked in many different psychiatric settings, from prisons to outpatient offices to medical and psychiatric hospitals. These days I work as an inpatient psychiatrist on the locked wards of a freestanding psychiatric hospital. I wrote the book not as a sequential exploration of patients I have encountered over these years but rather as a visiting and revisiting of hard questions that emerged for me about patients, and medicine, and the mind. Questions that stayed with and gnawed at me. This book arose from psychiatry's mysteries and my own misgivings, from patients whose struggles I could not make sense of, from the doubts and queries that haunted me and kept me from sleep at night.

I t was in my current job working weekends on the wards of the psychiatric hospital that I met Joseph. On the weekends I cover an entire adult unit in the hospital, which means that on Saturday mornings I will have eighteen to twenty patients to see. Before I see them, I will have had a brief Friday sign-out on each patient from the weekday doctor. Sometimes this will be a conversation that spans a few minutes. Sometimes it is a phrase written beside a name: 'resolving paranoia', for example, or 'manic, assaultive'. The nurse in charge of the unit meets me when I arrive and gives me pertinent information from the last twenty-four hours: vital signs, the degree to which a patient is participating in the unit therapy and activity groups, whether a patient is eating and taking her medications, whether a patient appears to be withdrawing from alcohol or from drugs. The nurse will also pass along anything the staff has noticed, either worrisome or reassuring. It is in this early-morning session that I hear about who wandered out of whose room naked and confused, who has gone two days now without talking to himself, who remains suspicious about whether her medications are poisoned, who was caught with cigarettes.

If a patient has been admitted overnight on Friday, then I will have the record of his emergency-room evaluation, but I will be the first treating psychiatrist to see him. It will be up to me to learn how the patient ended up in the hospital and how his treatment on the unit should begin.

This was the case for Joseph. When I walked onto the unit and saw his name listed as a new patient, I pulled his chart from the rack and flipped to the ER assessment: '42-year-old man with a history of depression who was referred by his caseworker after becoming increasingly depressed, not eating or drinking, not leaving his house, etc. Patient engages minimally with interview. States he wishes he were dead, but denies plan or intent to kill himself. Patient has been on antidepressants for many years, but recent compliance is questionable'.

Because of Joseph's 'minimal engagement', there wasn't much additional information in the evaluation. Our records showed that he had been hospitalized here five times before, but his most recent prior hospitalization had been seven years earlier. That was before the hospital had adopted computerized records, which meant that Joseph's records were entirely contained in paper charts, and those were archived. They could be requested, but it would require several days to obtain them. I needed to begin treating him now.

From the nursing report, I learned that Joseph had arrived on the unit and gone straight to bed, where he had been asleep for the last six hours. When the report had concluded, I made my way to his room to see him. I knocked on his door, and no one answered. I pushed the door open gently and called, 'Joseph? I'm Dr Montross. Okay with you if I come in?' The room was dark; the curtains were drawn. I took a step in and immediately noticed the smell of a person who had not bathed in some time. As my eyes adjusted to the darkness, I could hear

Joseph snoring loudly. It wasn't unusual for me to find my patients asleep. I started rounding early. Some patients, like Joseph, would have come to the hospital or would have been transferred from another ER in the middle of the night. Not infrequently, at some point in the admission process, patients received medication that had the potential to sedate them. I tried again.

'Joseph?' The snores continued. I turned and left the room. I'd give him some time to rest while I saw the other patients. If he hadn't woken up by the time I came back, I'd have to awaken him. For now I'd let him sleep.

I made my way around the unit, stopping into rooms to talk with the patients. I jotted down notes as to how they felt they were doing. I made myself a list of orders to write: medication changes for certain patients, additional privileges – like outdoor walks or permission to use their own razors – for others. I had met with about half the patients when Henry, an experienced nurse, pulled me aside, looking concerned.

'Hey, Doc,' Henry said. 'We've been trying to get Joseph up for his vitals. He's not responding at all. I even gave him a sternal rub, and nothing. Can you come over and examine him?'

I work with Henry frequently. He is easygoing and typically unflappable. Patients like him, I think in part because his demeanor is so even. Their worlds might feel chaotic, but Henry radiates calm. At this moment, however, he was talking quickly, and his tone was businesslike – a departure from his usual slow, unruffled jocularity. I took note immediately and followed him back across the unit toward Joseph's room. As we walked, Henry anticipated all my questions.

'I brought in the pulse ox and the manual cuff. His vitals are fine: one-eighteen over seventy-six, pulse of sixty-four. Oxygen saturation is ninety-eight percent on room air. But he's totally unresponsive. I checked the admission paperwork,' he continued. So had I. 'He blew a zero on the Breathalyzer when he came in, and he got no meds at all in the ER. He's been with us eight or nine hours now, and he was at least with it enough to register and get oriented to the unit on the night shift without them worrying he had a heavy dose of anything on board.' We got to the door, and Henry paused. 'I really dug my knuckles into his sternum, Doc.'

Sternal rubs are a seemingly vicious part of a neurological examination. People respond to different stimuli at different levels of consciousness. When afraid and alone in a quiet house, a person might be aware of the tiniest sounds or movements: the freezer's hum, the click of a thermostat, or the whisper of a single leaf fluttering outside a window. Adrenaline hones our senses and renders them keener. In contrast, in the depths of sleep I may not notice my partner's leg brushing up against my own. She may hear our daughter's single cough; I may not. There is a range of awareness. And yet the body's response to pain is preserved in these depths, for reasons that are evolutionarily obvious. Even in the deepest dream, a burning ember on your skin would wake you.

A sternal rub consists of making your hand into a fist and grinding your knuckles into a person's sternum, or breastbone. Try it on yourself; it doesn't take much pressure until you want the feeling to stop. With patients who are sound asleep, or sedated, or feigning unconsciousness, doctors and nurses first try less painful means of rousing them. If the gentler methods yield no response, so-called painful stimuli like the sternal rub may be employed. When someone truly does not respond to painful stimuli, there may be real cause for medical concern.

Most of us, as patients, are not entirely forthcoming with our doctors. We overestimate our exercise and round down on our junk-food consumption when we talk with our primary-care doctors. I generally tell my dentist that I floss more regularly than I do. The crass conventional wisdom in the emergency room is to use a formula when calculating the 'true' amount of alcohol a person drinks: Ask patients how many drinks they have in a typical week. Then, if the patient is female, multiply the number by two. For men, triple it. For veterans, multiply the number by five.

The true state of the psychiatric patients I treat may be obfuscated by a range of factors. Drugs – of both prescription and street varieties – are far more likely to be involved with my patients than with nonpsychiatric patients. Mentally ill people may be less able to accurately recount the symptoms they are experiencing or the drugs or medicines they have taken. They may be paranoid or angry and, as a result, refuse to disclose information that is important for me to know about their care. They may also – as in the case of suicidal patients who have intentionally overdosed – be less inclined to be forthcoming about what may have brought about changes in their condition or mental state. A pediatrician friend once joked that treating babies and young children can be like practicing veterinary medicine, since the patients cannot fully communicate with you. Sometimes psychiatry is similar; my colleagues and I must attempt to deduce what is going on when patients' explanations do not – or cannot – help.

I knew so little about Joseph that I had to keep a broad range of possibilities in mind. And if a patient was not responding, emergent causes needed to be ruled out first. It was reassuring that Henry had reported normal vital signs. Patients who overdose on opiates or sedatives have suppressed respiratory rates – they take fewer breaths per minute than a nonsedated person would, and their oxygenation levels drop accordingly. Joseph's breathing rate was normal, and so was the level of oxygen in his blood. But other medical emergencies could cause an acute change in someone's ability to respond. A neurological exam – including response to painful stimuli – could help determine whether there was a physical cause in his brain. I needed to know whether Joseph could be having a stroke, for example, or an otherwise undetectable seizure.

'Joseph?' I called loudly as I stood by his bedside. He remained motionless in the bed. I took hold of his shoulder and shook it. 'Joseph, I need you to wake up now,' I said. There was no response. Not even the snoring I had heard from him earlier in the morning. 'Okay, I'm going to examine you, Joseph,' I said as I lifted his limbs one by one from the bed. His reflexes were normal. I lifted his eyelids and shined a light in his eyes; his pupils were the same size, and they shrank in diameter when the light struck them. All reassuring signs. I began thinking that maybe Joseph was ignoring me, simply refusing to engage. Then I remembered Henry's sternal rub. I took Joseph's hand in mine and held my pen crosswise against his thumbnail. Then I pushed down on it, first gingerly and then, when there was no response from Joseph, as hard as I could. He didn't even flinch. The sensation of hard plastic pressing against a nail bed is unpleasant at best, excruciating at worst. Before a clinical-skills exam in medical school, I practiced it on my partner, Deborah, right after assessing her cranial nerves and position sense. Not having expected what was coming, she almost punched me. Joseph's lack of response was meaningful. It made me nervous. I started to leave the room, resolved that I would send Joseph out to a medical emergency room, but then turned back to him to try one last thing.

Doctors have tests that are specifically designed to determine whether symptoms are truly neurological in origin or whether they might have psychiatric or volitional components. Some of these tests are meant to flush out people who are exaggerating symptoms for their own gain. Disability applicants, perhaps, or military draftees. Many of these tests take advantage of basic tenets of brain functioning that are likely unknown to the general public. For example, in all but the most profound losses of cognitive functioning, people who sustain a brain injury will retain elementary facts: that a dog has four legs, for example, or that the date of Christmas is December 25. Even people with near-total memory loss know their own names. Answers to the contrary raise a flag of concern for malingering or symptom exaggeration.

Dr Charles Scott, a well-known forensic psychiatrist, demonstrates the coin-in-the-hand test to uncover intentionally erroneous responses on testing. 'You can't imagine that anyone would fall for this,' he says. 'It's very obvious.' Scott puts a coin on his desk and then puts his hands out in front of him, palms up, facing the person he's evaluating. Then he explains to the examinee that he's going to ask him or her to select which hand the coin is in. With the person watching, Scott picks up the coin with his right hand, slowly puts it in the palm of his left hand, and closes both of his hands into fists. The hands never cross; they are never out of the person's sight. 'That's it,' Scott says. Then, with all that in plain view, the examinee is asked to count down from ten to one and then say which hand the coin is in. Ninety-plus percent of non-malingering examinees will indicate the correct hand, Scott explains. Malingerers, conversely, will choose the wrong hand more than 50 percent of the time. They're trying too hard to look as if they can't function.

There are similarly cunning tests to assess pain, sensory loss, and paralysis. And as I turned away from Joseph, I suddenly remembered the arm-drop test. I stepped back to his bedside and raised his limp arm up above him until it was over his face. Then I let it drop. The arm flopped down, landing alongside Joseph's body. I did it again, raising the limb, holding it directly above and in line with his face, then letting it drop. Again the arm flopped to Joseph's side. Henry and I exchanged glances. The fact that Joseph's hand had missed hitting his face – twice – made it likely that he was changing the trajectory of his arm to protect himself. He may have been doing it unintentionally or subconsciously, but if he were totally unconscious he would have been unable to redirect his arm.

A group of internal-medicine doctors rotates through the psychiatric hospital early on weekend mornings to do physical exams on newly admitted patients and consultations for psychiatric patients who are medically complicated. I left Joseph's room and told Henry that I was going to page the medical service to run this by them. Now that I had seen the results of Joseph's arm-drop test, there was nothing else on exam that made me think he needed to be sent out to a medical hospital. Still, the lack of response to painful stimuli was unnerving. Henry agreed.

When I got the medical doctor on the phone, he had already left the hospital. 'Did you check his pupils?' he asked me. Yes, I told him, and his reflexes. And his muscle tone. Everything was normal except Joseph's lack of reaction to pain and the fact that he seemed to be protecting his face from his falling hand. The doctor listened, then thought aloud, ruling out one medical cause after another based on my examination. Eventually he paused. 'What about the gag?' he asked. 'Did you check a gag?' I hadn't. Lack of a gag reflex could indicate damage to the medulla, a critical part of the brain stem.

'I'll try it now,' I said.

'Call me if you need me,' the doctor replied. I hung up and headed back to Joseph's room with gloves and a tongue depressor. Henry met me in the doorway.

'Still nothing, Doc,' he said. 'I don't like it, but then again, he doesn't *seem* that sick to me.' I understood. Joseph's motionless endurance of two painful tests was impressive, but it didn't add up. I put on my gloves and went back to the bedside.

'Joseph?' I said loudly. 'I'm going to open your mouth to test your reflexes. This might feel uncomfortable. You might feel like you have to gag.' He remained stock-still and silent on top of his covers. I took his face in my hands and gently pulled his jaw open. I began to slide the tongue depressor into his mouth. Well before I was close to making him gag, Joseph let out a low moan. I paused and glanced up at Henry, who looked surprised. I withdrew the tongue depressor.

'Joseph?' I said again. 'Can you hear me?' The room was silent as Henry and I craned forward to listen for several long seconds. I began to convince myself that I had heard nothing and started to take Joseph's chin back into my hands. Then, finally, there came the slightest of sounds from his lips.

'*I'm very depressed,*' he whispered, motionless and eyes closed.

I suddenly heard myself exhale, relieved by Joseph's response. 'Okay,' I replied. 'Okay. We had some trouble waking you up and had to make sure you were with us.'

'I know where I am,' Joseph whispered, slowly and laboriously, 'and I know who you are, and I just want to be left alone, because I'm terribly depressed.'

It's tempting in situations like Joseph's to read a patient's lack of responsiveness as intentionally obstructionist, a manipulative trick. And yet the intersections between mind and body are so much deeper and more complex than that. My interpretation of Joseph's condition was that he had symptoms of catatonia.

Though catatonia is most widely associated with images of schizophrenic patients who adopt bizarre postures for prolonged periods of time, unresponsiveness and a lack of withdrawal from painful stimuli are indicative of stupor, a principal feature of catatonia.

Stupor illuminates a baffling intersection of the mind and body. Here psychic conflict can somehow interrupt a body's neural circuitry so as to render a person mute, immobile, or even impervious to pain. Psychiatry occupies just this kind of ever-shifting nexus of brain and mind. In terms of scientific disciplines, psychiatry bridges the territory between neurology and psychology. Like neurology (and unlike psychology), psychiatry is a medical discipline; practitioners of both disciplines must go to medical school, then train in a hospital-based residency program.

Neurology claims the territory of the brain, the spinal cord, and the nerves that branch throughout our bodies. The neurologist treats the migraineur whose headaches will not abate, the stroke victim who comes into the emergency room slurring her words and unable to move an arm and a leg, the boy who dives into the shallow end of the pool and becomes a quadriplegic, the motorcyclist whose crash has left him comatose from a bleeding brain.

Psychiatry, in contrast, is the science of disorders of the mind: when thoughts derail, emotions wreak havoc, or behavior destroys. In this book I have written five chapters about the mind and its mysteries. The first explores the struggles that doctors face in treating patients who intentionally and repeatedly injure themselves, by swallowing dangerous objects or by cutting and burning their own flesh; who undermine the very work their doctors do to try to help them. The second examines illnesses in which people are relentlessly tormented by their ideas about their bodies. Herein is a woman who nearly killed herself by picking at a blemish on her neck and a man whose earnest plea is for a surgeon to amputate his healthy leg. The third chapter centers on the legal ability doctors have to hospitalize – and sometimes medicate – a patient against his or her will. A patient claims that love emanates from everything around him. Is it ecstasy or psychosis? Do our current views of sanity allow for the otherworldly or divine experiences historically associated with saints or mystics? The fourth chapter grapples with the very real peril that patients face if their individual illnesses are not correctly defined. When a woman is admitted with repetitive thoughts of harming her child, her course of treatment – and her child's safety – depend upon whether she receives the correct diagnosis. The fifth and final chapter recalls Joseph and patients like him whose bodies are overtaken by the illnesses of their minds. How do we treat a woman whose seizures have no neurological cause? What possible explanation can there be when groups of men are convinced that their penises are shrinking into their bodies? The chapter asks how well we doctors, trained to act and fix, are prepared to sit with patients in – and accompany them through – the trials of their illnesses.

Life, of course, changes how we see things. As I wrote this book, my partner, Deborah, and I were raising our young daughter and our even younger son. It turns out that parenting children and caring for psychiatric patients have their fair share of similarities. I mean that in all the ways in which that sentence can be interpreted: with love, and frustration, and gratification. With fear, and awe, and ineptitude.

My children do not age sequentially in this book. My daughter may be four, and then she may be a newborn. I have found that I experience the pasts of my children in this jumbled way. A snapshot of a year ago and then a flowing current of their infancies and then today, with their book bags and lunch boxes and shoes that tie. I imagine that the memories will intermingle like this throughout their lives. Those memories, too, will shift with context. My son will become an engineer, and we'll nod knowingly, claiming to have seen it coming from the years of infinite Lego structures. Or he'll be a comedian and we'll say, *We knew because he always made his sister laugh*. Hindsight is powerful in parenthood, as in medicine.

I n its quest for effective treatments of mental illness, the evolution of psychiatry has been characterized by both inspiring and inglorious moments.

The Bethlem Hospital to which twenty-two-year-old Charles Harold Wrigley was admitted in 1890 was founded as a priory in 1247. It became a hospital in 1330 and took the first patients classified as 'lunatics' in 1357, making it the first and oldest recognized institution in the world to give care to the mentally ill. By the end of the fourteenth century, the hospital began to be used exclusively as a hospital 'for the insane'. Over the centuries the hospital grew, as did the demand for the care it provided. But for nearly three hundred years, Bethlem housed only twenty patients at a time and operated as an institution for so-called short-stay patients.

Today my colleagues and I use this term for hospital admissions whose duration is less than forty-eight hours. In the current state of health care in the United States, only the most severely ill patients are admitted to the hospital; even then the average stay is five days. Managed-care companies will phone physicians, sometimes daily, to interrogate them about their clinical decisions and treatment plans. If the insurance companies do not feel that the patient continues to meet their own narrow criteria for inpatient treatment, they will refuse to authorize additional days of hospitalization. Physicians have the right – indeed the mandate – to make clinical decisions based on patients' needs rather than insurance companies' pressures, but we are aware that unauthorized days in the hospital will result in staggering bills for our patients, many of whom are already in financial turmoil. If patients cannot pay, the costs of their treatments are frequently absorbed by the hospitals themselves – an obviously unsustainable practice. These factors combine to form the present reality: Today's inpatient care is most often crisis management. Patients are discharged from our wards as soon as they begin to stabilize, once they are no longer acutely psychotic or no longer in imminent danger of harming themselves or others. This means that patients are often released from the hospital in a tenuous state of mental healing. In many cases their symptoms recur and they return to the hospital for another five-day effort at stabilization.

In contrast, by early Bethlem standards a 'short stay' was one in which the patient was discharged after twelve months or less. Even one year of treatment proved to be inadequate for many patients at Bethlem, as the hospital archives reveal. The hospital developed a means of classifying patients as either 'curable' or 'incurable'.

'When a patient, after sufficient trial, is judged incurable', an eighteenth-century hospital document explains, 'he is dismissed from the hospital, and if he is pronounced dangerous either to himself or others, his name is entered into a book, that he may be received . . . [into] the house whenever a vacancy shall happen.' Despite the dangerous conditions that these patients were deemed to have, the number of patients in need of longer-term care far exceeded what Bethlem Hospital could offer. 'There are generally more than two hundred upon . . . the incurable list', the document continues, 'and as instances of longevity are frequent in insane persons, it commonly happens that the expectants are obliged to wait six or seven years, after their dismissal from the hospital, before they can be again received.'

In response to this great need, Bethlem expanded yet again in 1730, adding two wings for the 'incurables', who were now permitted to stay until the moment when – or if – they recovered. One such patient was Richard Dadd, an artist who began suffering from paranoid delusions at the age of twenty-five. Dadd said he received messages from the Egyptian god Osiris and stabbed his father to death in a park, believing him to be the devil in disguise. The hospital documentation mentions that Dadd remained in Bethlem until his death, forty-two years after he was first admitted to the incurable ward.

The expansion of Bethlem Hospital to treat – or at least contain – patients whose struggle with mental illness would be chronic and severe was not one entirely characterized by altruism. The sheer number and concentration of (often visibly) ill patients at Bethlem became a major eighteenth-century London tourist attraction. Visitors bought tickets from the hospital to gawk at the spectacles of both frenzied psychosis and the brutal forms of physical restraint that Bethlem employed. The tour began on the Bethlem grounds beneath two reclining sculpted figures called *Melancholy* and *Raving Madness* and then processed past the patients, some caged or shackled or with iron bits protruding from their mouths. Using Bethlem's name, the witnessing public soon coined a new word for the conditions they observed: 'bedlam'.

In retrospect, 'bedlam' seems an apt description both for the scenes of madness in Bethlem's early halls and for the torturous range of 'therapeutic' treatments whose efficacy was tested on the captive patients. Every spring, under the orders of one particular physician, there was a prescribed bloodletting for every patient in the hospital. At other times, depending on the psychiatric treatment currently in vogue, patients were restrained in submersible cages and then held underwater in the hopes that the near-drowning experience would shock the ill mind into a new outlook on life; they were strapped to seats that spun for hours at great speed, and treating practitioners marveled at how well the induced nausea would calm the most agitated patients into more placid behavior.

Even in that earlier era, a patient's finances could determine the treatment he received. Bethlem's eighteenth-century hospital physician, Thomas Monro, was called before a House of Commons committee to discuss the use of Gothic fetters – iron restraints to which hospitalized patients were frequently riveted. Monro reassured the committee that the fetters were 'fit only for the pauper lunatics', explaining that 'if a gentleman was put in irons, he would not like it'.

Though the treatments I can offer to my patients today are, thankfully, far more humane than those I find documented as I page through the nineteenth-century Bethlem casebooks, I am struck by the disquieting fact that Charles Harold Wrigley, with his exact symptoms and story, might as easily have been seen in one of the psychiatric wards on which I work today.

I could likely guarantee Mr Wrigley more dignity, more comfort, and more privacy than he received in 1890 in 'Bedlam'. I could prescribe him modern medications and offer him appropriate psychotherapy. But in spite of the surefire treatments that have been found in the last three centuries for countless *other* medical conditions, I could not guarantee that my treatment would bring him relief or cure.

So, standing in the dark of Joseph's room, my mind returned to young Charles Wrigley, who was described as miserable and holding his hand on his forehead as if in pain. 'I just want to be left alone,' Joseph had labored to tell me from his impenetrable stillness when I began to test his gag reflex. 'I'm terribly depressed.'

I sat down beside Joseph to ask him more questions, now that he'd broken his silence. 'How long have you been feeling this way?' I asked. His eyes remained closed. He did not respond.

'Joseph?' I tried again. 'I'd like to hear about what you've been going through so that I can help.' He did not stir. I sat there beside him, the awkward silence in the wake of my voice hanging between us. I felt a palpable discomfort – my own inability to penetrate Joseph's misery, the paralysis of his suffering. I found myself thinking of a short-lived flirtation I'd had with Buddhism in graduate school, when I'd sit and reach for the meditative stillness the practice espoused only to find my mind wandering and waylaid, my body stiff or itching. 'Joseph?' I said again. 'Joseph?' Eventually I stood and left the room.

Medicine asks its practitioners to confront the messy, unsatisfying, nonconforming human mind. As psychiatrists, we see the mind while it careens and lists, and we are not always sure how – or whether – we can right it. How do we respond when a patient's suffering breeds unbearable discomfort and unease within our own selves? What do we do when our patients' symptoms do not relent? When their experiences cannot be accounted for – or helped by – what we know about medicine, or the brain? *What then?*

CHAPTER ONE

The Woman Who Needed a Zipper

Those wounds heal ill that men do give themselves.

— Shakespeare, *Troilus and Cressida*

'Lauren's back again.' The gastroenterology fellow groaned. 'Lightbulbs this time.' I was in my second year of medical residency training and had just started working in a major medical hospital as a psychiatric consultant for medical and surgical inpatients. I had no idea who the fellow was talking about. When I told him so, he began to laugh. 'Oh, my God. You've never seen Lauren? Every time she comes in, the ER docs call us and we call you guys. We all give our advice on how to treat her, but you know what she really needs?' I didn't. 'A zipper,' he said. 'See you in the ER.'

I was utterly confused. Lightbulbs? A zipper? Sounded more like supplies for a child's science project than relevant clinical information. My mind was spinning as I walked through the dingy hospital stairwell to the emergency room to meet Lauren. On the wall at the landing hung a faded hospital-benefit poster of a horse-drawn carriage in the snow and some lines from Robert Frost. When I walked by the poster, I was typically working an overnight shift, and so 'miles to go before

I sleep' had taken on a bleary, fluorescent-lit meaning quite detached from woods, 'lovely, dark and deep'. As I swiped my badge to go into the ER, the lines were still running through my head: *Between the woods and frozen lake / The darkest evening of the year.*

Lauren was in a room across from the nurses' station. The ER rooms had three walls; the 'fourth wall' was a pink-and-tan curtain that could be drawn for privacy or pulled back to enter or exit. Lauren's curtain was wide open, and a security guard in a navy uniform sat in a plastic chair at the foot of her bed. I took a look in as I walked by. Given the gastroenterology fellow's dramatic reaction to her presence, I expected her appearance to be notable. It wasn't. She was sitting glumly on the bed, upright, in a hospital johnny. She was thin. Her dirty blond hair was a little mussed. She was twenty-five, but she looked slightly older. Otherwise, there was not much about her that was remarkable. I continued walking by; I wanted to take a look at her chart before I went in.

As I pulled Lauren's chart from the nurses' station, one of the nurses seated there glanced at my name tag. CHRISTINE MONTROSS, M.D., it read. PSYCHIATRY.

'Aha!' The nurse smiled and in a singsong voice added, 'I know who you're here to see.'

'The woman in 2B?' I asked. 'You know her?'

The nurse nodded and laughed, surprised. 'You don't? I thought everybody knew Lauren. Have fun!' She winked and handed me a folder with the patient's ER paperwork in it. 'Oh, Doc?' she called as I walked away. 'Don't lend her that nice pen of yours.'

I opened the chart. A sheet of Lauren's orders was on top. Along with the ticked boxes indicating the conventional laboratory studies for ER patients were a few additional specifications: 'Finger food diet only', read one line. Beneath it: '**NO** objects to be left in room – SEE BEHAVIORAL CARE PLAN.' I couldn't be sure how to interpret these orders, but from them I surmised that Lauren must be either suicidal or homicidal. Patients who were relegated to finger-food diets were those who could not be trusted with utensils.

Beneath the orders page was a sheet of Lauren's lab values. I quickly scanned it, looking for the typical irregularities of psychiatric patients: elevated blood-alcohol levels, a positive drug test, subtherapeutic medication levels, thyroid abnormalities, infection. With the exception of a toxicology screen that was positive for her having smoked marijuana sometime recently, nothing stood out. Her complete blood count and electrolytes were totally normal. Her pregnancy test was negative. Chest and abdominal X-rays had been taken; the results were pending.

I flipped through the remainder of the paperwork and found that Lauren was already slated for admission to a bed on the internal-medicine service. The admitting house officer had seen her and written a note. I deciphered the scrawled shorthand to read: 'This patient is a well-known 25-year-old female with extensive psych history and multiple previous intentional ingestions.' Usually an 'intentional ingestion' meant that someone had drunk bleach or eaten rat poison or overdosed on pills as a suicide attempt, but the meaning was different here. Light-bulbs. Suddenly keeping utensils and objects and nice pens out of Lauren's reach made sense. Nobody wanted her to swallow them.

I walked past the security guard and into Lauren's room. Before I could introduce myself, she glared at me and said, 'Let me guess, you're the shrink, right? I can always tell you guys – you're all nicey-nice handshakes and dipshit smiles.' The security guard, who had doubtless seen a number of ER psych consults, stifled a chuckle and put his fist over his mouth to hide a grin.

'Sounds like you've pegged us,' I answered, reaching out my right hand in a nicey-nice shake. 'I'm Dr Montross.'

'Yeah,' replied Lauren, glowering at my hand without taking it. 'I can read your fuckin' name tag, *Christine,* but unless you are going to get me something for this pain, I'm not in the mood for a conversation.'

I turned to the security guard. 'Would you mind letting us talk alone for a minute?' I asked.

'Whatever you say, Doc.' He shrugged. 'I'll be right outside if you need me.' He stepped out and drew the curtain closed behind him when he left. I slid his chair to the side of Lauren's bed and sat down.

Lauren pulled the hospital blanket up to her neck, lay down against her pillow, and rolled onto her side, turning her back to me. 'Jesus, you people don't *listen*. I wasn't kidding. Unless you give me something for my pain, I'm not talking.'

'Since I'm meeting you for the first time, it's hard for me to know about your pain. If you tell me about it, maybe we can come up with a way I could be of help,' I offered. It was a stretch – she was talking physical pain, and I was going to try to access her psychic pain – but it didn't feel like a lie. I knew I wasn't going to write her an order for pain medication – that was the territory of the ER and the medicine teams – but I needed an entrée, and I hoped that asking about her pain would soften her defensive stance. Or at least encourage her to roll over and look at me. 'What's going on that you've ended up in the emergency room?'

'Read. The. Chart,' Lauren intoned, not making a move.

'I've looked at it a bit already,' I said, 'but I'd actually rather hear from you – '

'Well, I'd rather be left alone,' she interrupted.

'Fair enough,' I said. 'Let me just read you what I've got here, and you tell me whether that sounds about right, okay?' I opened the chart to the admission note. Lauren was silent. 'It says here that you were feeling upset and that you swallowed some pieces of a lightbulb. Is that right?'

Lauren scoffed, then abruptly turned toward me, angry. 'Yeah, "upset". That's one way to put it. See? That's why I don't talk to you people. I'm in the hospital three days ago, you all decide – you shrinks and the surgeons and the gastrointestinal docs – you all decide to kick me out even though I'm telling everybody *I'm not ready to go home,* and then some intern writes that I'm "upset". Well, fuck yeah, I'm upset. I'm upset because I told you I wasn't ready to go home and no one listened to me. So pardon me if I don't really buy that you're so *interested* in my side of things.'

'What happened with the lightbulb?' I asked.

'Lightbulbs,' she said.

'Okay, what happened with the lightbulbs?'

'I was pissed off. I crushed them up and swallowed them,' she said matter-of-factly. 'Not the metal part, just the glass and wire.' I nodded. There was a moment of quiet between us. Then she spoke. 'Now do you believe me that my stomach fucking hurts?'

I left Lauren and went off to write up my evaluation and recommendations. The surgical team to which she would be assigned consulted the psychiatry service for help in managing her psychiatric medications while she was hospitalized. The team's larger hope, of course, was that we would be able to provide some sort of intervention that would break the pattern of Lauren's swallowing, or at least lengthen the periods of time in between her intentional ingestions. To better understand the medications she had been on and the psychiatric treatments she had tried prior to this admission, I pulled her old charts from medical records. She had stacks of them, some of which were more than four years old and so had been archived. I looked up the most recent admissions that had taken place in the last four years; there were twenty-three. Her hospitalizations had been prompted by her ingestion of the following:

ninety screws
AA batteries and paper clips
two knife blades and four fork handles
four candles

four metal spoon handles
the screwdriver from an eyeglass-repair kit
a knife and six barbecue skewers
a bedspring
thirteen pencils
a knife, a knife handle, and a mercury thermometer
a box of three-inch galvanized nails
a screwdriver, a ninja knife, and a knife blade
a steak knife
a razor and five pens
two knives
scissors, pins, and a nail file
four four-inch pieces of curtain rod
scissors, a drill bit, and a pen
a six-inch piece of curtain rod and a seven-inch knife
a knife, three spoons, and some copper wire
two six-inch steak knives
a pair of scissors
a four-inch metal blade, three spoon handles, and a nail clipper

Over and over, Lauren would swallow potentially dangerous objects in the context of stress. She swallowed the screwdriver, the knife blade, and the ninja knife when she learned that her uncle was terminally ill. The two knife blades and four fork handles were a response to learning that her sister had hepatitis. The box of nails was after a fight with a neighbor. Each time she said she felt better after she had swallowed something and then brought herself to the emergency room for treatment. Over and over, doctors performed endoscopies, threading a camera and tools down Lauren's throat with a tube to try to get the objects out before the things she had swallowed inflicted damage on her esophagus, stomach, or intestines. Only once, after she'd ingested a single spoon handle, was endoscopy deemed unnecessary. 'She had some discomfort', the discharge summary read, 'but the spoon passed normally.'

In contrast, once, when an eight-inch knife blade was too dangerous to pull back up through her esophagus and out of her mouth, Lauren's abdomen had to be surgically opened and the knife removed. Many times, multiple endoscopic attempts were required to 'retrieve' the same object. One endoscopy note read, 'Four approximately 4-inch-long sharp pieces of broken curtain rail were found in the gastric fundus. Removal of two was accomplished with a snare. The other two could not be removed. They kept holding up at the gastroesophageal junction despite two hours' manipulation.' If objects could not be extracted, more experienced doctors were brought in for additional attempts. A senior physician developed a reputation for being able to retrieve items Lauren had swallowed when others had failed to do so. Once, during a hospital meeting that had specifically been convened to discuss Lauren's care, an administrator asked the gathered group of clinicians for ideas about a systematic approach for treating her during her recurrent admissions. A GI fellow piped up from the back, 'If at first you don't succeed, try, try again. If you still don't succeed, call in Dr Friedrichs.'

Not infrequently, once awake and recovering back on the floor, Lauren would swallow something in her hospital room and require further treatment. Several times she swallowed the handles of spoons from her meal trays. Once a pencil. Once she broke fragments of wood from the frame of her room's window and ate them. One night in the emergency room, she removed and swallowed a metal piece of the gurney.

The doctors charged with Lauren's care had no choice but to treat her when she came to the emergency room. Each time her actions were potentially life-threatening. To deny her care not only would be ethically incomprehensible but could also be medically catastrophic. No one could suggest that doctors should refuse to perform procedures on her, even if the procedures themselves were somehow reinforcing the maladaptive behavior, even if Lauren might swallow something as soon as she awakened from an endoscopy that had narrowly averted disaster. And yet the frustration of the surgical staff, who once during a consultation expressed their shared wish to 'let her experience the consequences', was only partially an emotional response to her flagrant self-injury and misuse of their expertise. It was also a manifestation of the fact that they felt they were contributing to this young woman's demise. 'It doesn't matter that she's the one that swallowed the razor,' one surgical house officer said to me. 'If I have to operate, I'm the one that's cutting her open, exposing her to the dangers of major surgery, giving her a belly full of scar tissue. . . . I might fix the emergency, but beyond that, none of what I'm doing is going to help her in the long run.'

Many surgeons differentiate their field of medicine from others by their ability to perform a procedure that fixes what's wrong with the patient. Surgeons realign the broken hip and remove the cancerous breast; they repair gunshot wounds and replace burned skin. One particularly brazen surgeon with whom I trained as a medical student would routinely wait for his patients to awaken from anesthesia and then come to the bedside, look them in the eye, and announce, 'I cured you!' This was all the more disquieting to observe given that some of his patients were terminally ill, and his role – to remove a cancer-ridden lobe of the liver or extricate a tumor-infested loop of bowel – might well have been only palliative in nature.

In general, the surgeons with whom I work have a great respect and appreciation for the field of psychiatry, but they also feel they'd be particularly ill suited to practice it. Lauren was an unsettling patient for all of us, but psychiatrists often face complex patients and ambiguous diagnoses. Lauren's condition was particularly irritating for the surgeons who treated her. The chronic, 'unfixable' nature of her illness was made plain in her personalized Medical and Behavioral Treatment Plan, the first line of which read, 'Approach for this patient should focus on disease management, not cure.'

By continuing to ingest objects in the hospital, Lauren was not only putting herself at risk but also putting her doctors and the hospital at risk. A hospital's job, by definition, is to keep patients safe and healthy. In the treatment of psychiatric patients, this means that reasonable measures must be taken to prevent potentially dangerous patients from having a way to hurt or kill themselves or others. For these very reasons, many psychiatric hospitals have specialty fixtures. Door handles and showerheads flip down when weight is put on them to prevent patients from hanging themselves. Beds and couches are often built into the walls to prevent them from being upended or used to blockade doors. Patients on 'suicide precautions' cannot shave with razors, nor are they permitted to have belts on their pants or laces in their shoes.

With Lauren, *everything* was theoretically ingestible. To protect her – and themselves – hospital administrators developed a Behavioral Care Plan specific to Lauren, outlining the 'Process for admission to [an] inpatient unit':

1. Immediate Security Constant Observation with **TWO** guards
2. Immediate sweep and removal of any and all objects inside patient room
3. Objects for removal are not limited to but must include:
    a. controls for blinds
    b. clock and batteries
    c. regular trash barrel and all bags
    d. biohazard container and bag
    e. all pens, pencils, markers, books, thumbtacks
    f. hygiene-related products (soap, toothbrush, toothpaste, mouthwash, powder, and all applicable containers, etc.)
    g. artwork
    h. wall hangings, clips, nails, and signs
    i. nonessential medical-related equipment

      j. any nonessential, non-medical-related items

      k. fan

      l. beverage containers/bottles

4. Patient is to receive finger foods ONLY.

      a. Meals delivered on a single Styrofoam plate/tray only.

      b. Beverages are to be given in a single Styrofoam cup with refills to occur outside patient room.

      c. Plastic or metal utensils are NOT allowed.

      d. Immediate removal of tray/plate when meal has been completed.

5. Staff must only bring essential items into room at point of care and remove once completed:

      a. IV poles, tubing, labels, fluid bags, flushes, etc.

      b. tape and/or dressing supplies, etc.

6. All new Constant Observers/Security Officers are to be educated by nurse about patient's status prior to entering room.

      a. All nonclothing objects are to be removed (badges, clips, keys, pens, etc.).

      b. Patient's mouth must be in view and observed at all times.

      c. Patient must have one arm visible above the sheets/blankets at all times.

      d. Patient is not allowed to hide mouth with gown, blanket, sheet, etc.

7. Patient may not leave designated room unless for an ordered test/procedure.

8. Patient must remain in hospital attire for her entire stay, undergarment briefs allowed, bathrobe belts/ties not allowed.

The implications of the list were startling to read. Styrofoam trays, plates, and cups prevented Lauren from breaking a ceramic plate or a plastic tray into jagged pieces to swallow. Even bringing a plastic bottle or pitcher into the room to refill her drink posed a risk. If curtain rods had been broken into sharp shafts and swallowed, then IV poles could be, too. The costs of these admissions were also unquestionably staggering. Two guards had to be paid hourly for the entire hospitalization, simply to sit in Lauren's room and watch her.

As I turned the pages of her chart, I came across a range of surgical notes and consultations. Brief blurbs by surgical residents revealed that they had put the trauma surgery team on alert, in case one of Lauren's swallowed objects obstructed or perforated her gut, necessitating emergency surgery. Previous psychiatric consultations focused on the acuity of Lauren's mental state. Was she currently having urges to swallow objects or to otherwise hurt herself? Was she suicidal?

The pages of notes also delineated the psychiatric medications that Lauren had been prescribed prior to her admission and whether or not she'd been taking them reliably. At various times Lauren had been on medications from almost every class of psychopharmacologic agent: antidepressants and mood stabilizers, sedatives and antipsychotics. Frequently she was prescribed more than one at a time: an antidepressant to improve her mood and a sedative to treat her anxiety, for example. During one series of admissions, the plan was to target her impulsivity with a mood stabilizer and an antipsychotic that had recently shown promise for behavioral dyscontrol in a clinical trial. Judging from the frequency of Lauren's admissions and the similarity of her symptoms on arrival, no specific medication seemed to make much of a difference.

All of medicine is plagued by the whims of the body and the variability of the human experience. The most effective diabetes regimen is useless if the patient to whom it is prescribed binges on candy bars and soda. A vegan marathoner may still have stubbornly high cholesterol or be genetically predisposed to coronary artery disease. Psychiatry's particular struggle is that it is so often impossible to separate our patients' psychiatric symptoms from the social circumstances and stressors that exacerbate them. There are many frustrating consequences of this dilemma.

A common critique of psychiatry is that our medications do not work or that, if they do, they only subdue and sedate. This misperception has sometimes led psychiatry to be cast as a sinister science, beholden to pharmaceutical companies that wish to unnecessarily medicate the masses for profit. The antipsychiatry movement perpetuates this characterization of psychiatry as a scienceless discipline. Dr Thomas Szasz, a famed critic of psychiatry who happened to be a psychiatrist himself, deemed the field 'pseudoscience' and likened it to alchemy and astrology. Scientology has taken particular aim at psychiatry (as Tom Cruise demonstrated in his cruel and absurd rants against the existence of postpartum depression), even funding a hyperbolically named 'museum' in California called Psychiatry: An Industry of Death.

Dr Lawrence Price, my friend and mentor who has been at the forefront of the study of mood disorders for thirty years, more appropriately identified some of the issues that give rise to mistrust of psychopharmacology in a 2010 letter to the editor of the *New York Times*. 'Antidepressants do work for people who are really depressed', he writes. 'They don't for people who aren't. Depression is frequently diagnosed in people who don't have it, and frequently not diagnosed in those who do. Medications that work for depression are commonly misused, and types of psychotherapy that work for depression are commonly not used at all. The reasons for this state of affairs include mistrust of authority, stigma, big-stakes health care economics, cross-discipline rivalries and simplistic thinking (within the mental health care field as well as the general public). The excesses of the media and the perverse incentives of our current health care delivery system make things worse.'

Dr Price was writing specifically about the treatment of depression, but the obstacles he identifies are germane to the current treatment of most psychiatric illnesses. As I looked through the long list of psychiatric medications that Lauren had tried – and that had failed to improve her condition – I found that many of these confounding variables were at play. It was possible that medication *could* be of help to Lauren. Depression or anxiety could underlie her swallowing. If those illnesses were treated, she might be more able to cope in healthy ways when she was distressed. And yet even the most perfect medications cannot help if they are not reliably taken. Some of the notes indicated that Lauren had run out of her medication and lacked the means to obtain more. Others reported that she had discontinued a treatment regimen because she found the side effects intolerable. Still others mentioned that she had been drinking or using drugs that had the potential to interfere with her medications.

Nearly every note made mention of Lauren's 'lack of coping mechanisms', as well as a litany of seemingly insurmountable social stressors – poverty, unemployment, family discord, lack of social supports. No pill we could prescribe would address any of these issues, all of which were constant pressures upon Lauren in her daily outpatient life.

In Lauren's charts, interspersed between the consultations and the daily progress notes by her medical team, were the images from her many, many endoscopies: healthy tubes of bright pink flesh that terminated in a glint of metal knife blade or the white plastic cap of a give-away pen.

Under normal circumstances, when endoscopic procedures yield biopsies or polyps that have been removed from the body's depths, these specimens are sent to the hospital's pathology department for description and evaluation. Lauren's specimens followed protocol. A surgical pathology report: 'Received fresh' – as opposed to in formalin, as would be true for many anatomical specimens – 'are silver metal, focally rusted scissor blades with a small amount of attached orange plastic handle. The specimen measures 14.3 × 3.0 × 0.8 cm.' As if to justify the fact that the pathologist had not microscopically evaluated the scissors, the report continues, 'Gross diagnosis only, consistent with foreign body.'

This terminology, 'foreign body', crops up again and again in the medical assessment of Lauren. Each time she comes to the hospital, X-rays are done, to enable us both to look at what is inside her and where and to make sure that none of it has perforated the critical barrier between the messy, bacteria-laden contents of the human gut and the sterile body cavity that holds our internal organs. 'Foreign body in the stomach/esophagus', reads a typical abdominal X-ray report in Lauren's chart, '14 cm in greatest dimension. Multiple other small foreign bodies, unspecified'.

The language is meant not to be evocative but rather efficiently dichotomous. Classifying an object on a medical image as 'foreign' is a way of differentiating self from other. A child inhales a button, or a game piece, or a nickel, and a 'foreign body' is visible in the airway on a chest X-ray.

There are sometimes objects that are *of* the body that nonetheless don't belong: a cyst, a tumor. Yet as much as my mother might have thought of her breast cancer as an invader, as something 'other' than her body, the cells were her own, built by her DNA, errant as it might have been. Neither the unwelcome tumor in her breast nor the cancerous cells in her axillary lymph node – despite their unmistakable invasion of her healthy tissue – could medically be classified as 'foreign'.

And yet in describing Lauren's medical and psychiatric plight, this recurrent phrase – 'foreign body' – seemed profoundly correct. Was there some way in which Lauren was disconnected from her body? Some separation that enabled her to swallow scissors and steak knives?

Most of us are unable to intentionally inflict injury upon ourselves, let alone understand what would lead someone to do so. This may be because of a reflexive response to pain or the result of an innate survival drive. It may be because our sense of personhood is so inextricably tied to our bodies that it is often impossible for us to separate our identities from our physical selves. Self-injury is even less comprehensible to us than suicide. Suicide at least can be cast as a desperate attempt to end torment and pain. How do we make sense of behavior whose very intention is to *bring about* damage and pain and yet survive? Over and over in Lauren's chart, she describes swallowing objects in an attempt to relieve stress, not as a means of killing herself. Though she does occasionally express thoughts of wanting to die, those instances are very rare in comparison to the relentless constancy of her dangerous ingestions.

What, then, is this disconnect in Lauren and in others like her who chronically and persistently struggle with what psychiatry calls 'non-suicidal self-injury'? Why is it that simply reading about the wounds she has inflicted upon herself causes many of us to wince (barbecue skewers? a bedspring?), while Lauren and others who chronically harm themselves not only can tolerate inflicting these actions upon themselves but may indeed find some sort of *relief* in doing so? Could it be that her body is not inseparable from her sense of self but rather foreign to it?

D r Armando Favazza is a leading expert on self-mutilation. Favazza, a professor of psychiatry at the University of Missouri, developed a system for categorizing deviant self-harm. He classified self-injurious behavior as falling into one of three types: major, stereotypic, or superficial/moderate.

Major self-mutilation comprises rare and extreme cases – people who, for example, cut off their own limbs, castrate themselves, enucleate their eyes. These patients are most often psychotic. They may be commanded to act by hallucinations or religious delusions; they may feel they have been explicitly instructed by God to harm themselves. There are multiple references in the psychiatric literature to people who have removed one of their eyes, citing a passage in the biblical book of Matthew in which Jesus commanded, 'If thy right eye offend thee, pluck it out.' Deliberate eye mutilation is a severe act, but it is not altogether uncommon. Favazza estimates that in the United States alone, about five hundred cases of intentional eye enucleation occur every year.

Many episodes of major self-injury – whether to eyes or other parts of the body – are in response to sexual perseverations or themes. In *Bodies Under Siege,* Favazza describes an example reported in the *Journal of Clinical Psychiatry* by J. E. Crowder in which a forty-four-year-old man tried to gouge out his eyes with his fingers because he felt guilty for having gone to topless nightclubs. Three years after this first attempt, he felt that a statue of the Virgin Mary commanded him to remove his eyes from his body and thus cleanse himself of sin. He attempted to do so, this time using forceps. He failed and was psychiatrically hospitalized, where he repeatedly tried to take out his eyes, eventually succeeding in jamming a pencil into one of them during psychological testing.

Examples abound in religious literature of men who, having failed in their strivings to attain purity through abstinence, castrate themselves. Interestingly, very few documented cases of psychopathological female genital self-mutilation exist. Though insertion of all manner of objects into the vagina is not uncommon, Favazza reports that there are only six cases in the psychiatric literature in which mentally ill women have intentionally mutilated their own genitals.

Which does not mean that women do not grievously and graphically harm themselves in other ways. I recently treated a middle-aged psychotic woman who repeatedly injured herself, believing that her suffering was penance and had been mandated by God. She was sent from a medical emergency room to the psychiatric hospital because her torso was covered with blistered burns from cigarettes that she had ground into her skin. Obtaining information from her was difficult because she spoke of herself in the third person, as if the voice coming from her lips were God's. 'I have allowed Patty to afflict her body in my service,' she would intone. 'I have granted her the gift of doing penance, and you see the results before you.' Then she would seamlessly segue into describing why one of the other patients – in this case, a highly anxious young man with a tendency toward paranoia who kept looking fearfully at Patty – had been chosen as her 'supreme pope' and under whose hospital bed she claimed her cat, Daffodil, was hiding. It was only after a lengthy interview, which required me to constantly redirect Patty's God-voiced proclamations, that she revealed to me she had inserted scissors into her rectum and 'opened and closed them at every station of the cross'. I sent her back to the medical hospital, where a sigmoidoscopy revealed multiple internal lacerations.

Favazza notes that not all acts of self-mutilation classified as major are committed by patients in the throes of psychosis. Some may occur in states of drug- or alcohol-induced intoxication. Heartbreaking accounts exist of men who have amputated their penises or testicles as a result of being tormented by their homosexual desires. Episodes of self-castration or of breast amputation have been noted as desperate measures taken by transgender people.

One might think that the extremity of pain and danger inflicted by these wounds would shake even psychotic people into a state of alarm. In fact, the opposite is frequently true. Of people who commit major self-injury, Favazza has been quoted as saying that 'despite the severity of their wounds, [they] feel little pain at the time or regret afterward. . . . It is as if their action has resolved the conflict within them'.

In contrast to major self-mutilation, stereotypic self-mutilation occurs most frequently in the context of learning or developmental disability – in some forms of what has historically been called mental retardation, for example, or in more severe forms of autism. It may even occur in very severe forms of Tourette's disorder or obsessive-compulsive disorder, in which the sufferers tragically recognize the self-injury as irrational but are unable to refrain from carrying it out nonetheless. Patients who stereotypically harm themselves may rhythmically bang their heads, requiring protective helmets; they may hit or bite themselves. I treated one such patient who compulsively gouged and tore at her face, leaving angry wounds that festered and would not heal. Each time even a preliminary scab formed, the young girl would, once unattended, desperately claw at her cheek or lip or chin, reopening the wound.

The most common category of self-mutilation – with sufferers found across the globe and in every socioeconomic class – is the superficial/moderate type. Though Lauren's chronic swallowing of objects seems neither superficial nor moderate, it is into this group that she and her symptoms fall. In her company would be a comparatively tame crowd who compulsively pull their own hair, bite their nails, and scratch their skin. Others, with symptoms more analogous in severity to Lauren's, repeatedly cut and carve their skin, burn themselves, stick needles into their bodies, and break their own bones. Burning and cutting are the most common types of self-injury, with experts currently estimating that as many as 2 million Americans intentionally engage in those particular acts each year.

For many of these 2 million, occasional, episodic self-harm becomes progressively more frequent, reinforcing an unhealthy feedback loop in the brain. A person turns to self-injury, and the act of cutting or burning or swallowing provides a release. Not unlike what happens with a person who turns to drugs or alcohol in distress, an insidious pattern develops. It is for this that Favazza has described the behaviors associated with superficial/moderate self-injury as 'morbid forms of self-help'. Tracing the skin with a blade, holding flame to flesh, or, in Lauren's case, consuming something dangerous provides distraction from distress and relief from emotional discomfort. Yet this relief is impermanent. The distress returns, and without a lasting means of addressing the unease, Lauren and others like her continue to seek temporary reprieve in reenacting their rituals of self-harm.

If the feedback loop takes hold, Favazza explains, the harmful behaviors 'become an overwhelming preoccupation and are repeated over and over again', constituting what he has termed 'the repetitive self-mutilation syndrome'. People with this syndrome may truly feel as though self-injury is an addiction, and in severe cases their pattern of turning to it in times of distress may last for decades. Even when it remits, it is typically not without consequence. Favazza describes the 'normal course' of repetitive self-mutilation syndrome as 'ten to fifteen years during which the self-mutilation is interspersed with periods of total quiescence [as well as periods of] impulsive behaviors such as eating disorders, alcohol and substance abuse, and kleptomania'.

For family members and clinicians who care for self-injurers, the act of self-harm is frequently incomprehensible and the impulsivity associated with it can be infuriating. The primary response evoked in caregivers is often one of anger and resentment. After I first saw Lauren, I went from the emergency room up to the hospital floor where she was to be admitted so that I could see the preparations taking place for her admission. Nurses and other staff members were busily removing medical equipment from the walls, taking away all loose objects, and covering over fixtures. I stood in the doorway. The only other times I had seen this many hospital employees in a patient room, a code had been called because someone was in cardiac arrest and needed resuscitation.

'Wow,' I said astutely.

A nurse walked by me, carrying parts of a metal IV pole. 'Yeah, wow,' she said with a sarcastic snort. 'As if I'm not busy enough, I gotta waste time pulling all this apart for our most frequent flier every time she decides she wants a little attention. It's not like there are other patients of mine who are . . . I don't know, actually *sick* or something. God forbid I spend my time doing things for them."

As the nurse passed, I stood there, amazed at the chaos that one person's self-directed actions could cause. Each time Lauren swallowed a potentially dangerous object, she wielded her power to cause institutional upheaval and widespread personal disequilibrium. She angered nurses and surgeons; she sent administrators into flurries of paperwork; she prompted special case conferences and grand-rounds debates; she ignited infighting between medical disciplines eager to disclaim primary responsibility for her care. While hospitalized, she was rude and unappreciative at best, provocative and hostile at worst. She cost people time and money and patience. During one particular period, there was even a superstitious policy among house officers: They refused to say Lauren's name aloud, lest doing so should conjure her to appear in the emergency room later that shift.

I was not immune to Lauren's maelstrom. Once she was admitted, I visited her room daily, attempting to engage her in any way I could. I tried to connect with her, at first naïvely and pridefully, hoping I could penetrate her caustic exterior and, in doing so, truly steer her toward health. During one visit I tried to offer her a chance to talk about the experiences that had led to her behaviors; during the next I proposed that we discuss coping strategies she could utilize when she felt the urge to swallow something. Despite the lengthy list of medications she'd tried, I went through them one by one with her, struggling in vain to discern whether any one of them had been more helpful than another. Each time I saw her, I endeavored to cajole her into seeing the benefit she would reap from committing more fully to the outpatient treatment that she would have after she was discharged. Perhaps, I imagined, my empathetic ear could succeed where so many others had failed. This fantasy, of course, was fleeting. Some days she ignored me; others she tore into me in a fit of rage.

Lauren met each of our encounters with derision. Although I typically felt composed and in control during clinical meetings with patients, working with Lauren made me feel inept. I couldn't even reasonably call it 'working with Lauren'. I was floundering, and I was sure she could see it. No matter how steadily I attempted to keep my cool, I began to feel that Lauren could sniff out my discomfort. As a psychiatrist, I felt confident in my ability to make patients feel calm and safe in my presence. But Lauren's turmoil wouldn't steady. Rather than providing her with security, I felt as though I were absorbing her unease. And the more wobbly I felt, the more emboldened and unwavering her aggressive stance became. My savior fantasies vanished, and I began to dread my daily obligation to round on her.

One day Lauren was particularly nasty to me. Early in my psychiatric training, I learned that mentally ill people can harbor an uncanny ability to detect – and then broadcast – a person's most exquisitely sensitive vulnerabilities. During my first week as a psychiatry house officer, I shuddered as an agitated, psychotic woman screamed a series of vile racial epithets and accusations at the security guards who had restrained her and were carrying her to the seclusion room. A month or two later, I treated a demented man who routinely approached a nurse who, unbeknownst to him, was a rape survivor; he ranted through a litany of aggressive and explicit sexual acts he said he intended to force upon her while she slept. A friend and colleague of mine, besieged by guilt after his depressed mother committed suicide, had a therapy patient who knew nothing about the death and yet began leaving my friend daily voice-mail messages saying that she was going to kill herself and, if she did, that it would be my friend's fault because he did not save her.

A mentally ill person's accuracy in hitting the mark could be mere coincidence. Or there may be a kind of perceptual acuity that sharpens in the dangerous throes of madness, as hearing or eyesight might in a life-or-death chase. Without excluding those possibilities, I have come to think of this form of cruelty as a combination of disinhibition and powerlessness. The social filter that prevents a person from saying wildly inappropriate things can dissolve when the mind is sick. And any animal, when it perceives itself to be cornered and in mortal danger, desperately lashes out in the way most likely to make its aggressor retreat. And so in the cases of people who are psychiatrically ill, the ferocity is not so much a character trait of the person doling it out. The ferocity is rather a symptom, brought about by the stark territory of mental illness and its lonely, fearsome landscape.

In Lauren this vitriol came at me after days of the silent treatment. Dutifully, if halfheartedly, I knocked on her open door one late afternoon. 'Lauren? It's Dr – '

'I know who the fuck it is,' Lauren interrupted. She sat up and began to address the two security guards at her bedside, gesturing toward me. 'This fuckin' Amazonian joker comes in every day with her overgrown, ugly-ass eyebrows and talks to me like I'm a two-year-old just so she can feel like she's saving the world and write some bullshit nonsense in my chart about how my psych meds need to be changed.' My stomach – within my six-foot-tall frame with its badly untended eyebrows – dropped. *Had* I been condescending to her? *Had* I gotten carried away with narcissistic fantasies?

'She has no fuckin' clue what to do with me, so she goes all rich-girl-who-went-to-Brown, "Let's talk about some healthy ways to handle your feelings" so she can get out of here, dope me up on more of those horse pills, and tell everybody she's a fuckin' regular Dr Phil!' The guards looked toward me sheepishly for a response.

'Well . . . at least you're telling me how you feel,' I stammered, trying to gauge whether or not I was blushing. I wondered if Lauren and the guards all thought that I was as inept as she was making me out to be, as inept as I suddenly felt.

'"*At least you're telling me how you feel*,"' Lauren mocked in a whining singsong. 'Get the fuck outta my face, Amazon Brown.'

I felt both humiliated and relieved. She was giving me a way out. 'I'm not going to force you to talk to me, Lauren,' I replied.

'No, you sure as hell are not,' she shot back.

'But I really am trying to be helpful to you,' I said, turning to leave the room, 'and I'm happy to talk later if you're feeling more up to it.'

As I passed through the door, she let loose with a final arrow. 'Don't hold your breath. Maybe use the time instead to get you some tweezers.'

As I walked away, I heard one of the guards whistle softly and let out a giggling 'Damn!'

D uring my third year as a medical student, a notoriously demanding and demeaning surgical attending physician had gathered a group of us together to ask for feedback on our experience of the surgical clerkship. Though we had all found it both unnecessarily grueling and poorly organized, my peers dutifully offered enthusiastic praise as the attending went around the table, soliciting comments. When he reached me, last, I offered constructive criticism that was honest and fair. He was silent for a moment and then responded.

'I don't know what you've heard about how you'll be graded in this clerkship,' he began quietly, and then gestured to his shoes. 'But these are the feet that are connected to the legs that are connected to the ass that you should be kissing right now.' He paused for effect, then continued. 'Do you want to rethink your feedback?'

At the time I was deeply humiliated *and* enraged. Yet by now I had all but forgotten about him. However, in the midst of my treatment of Lauren, I had a dream that I was a medical student again, assisting that same antagonistic surgeon in an operation. In the dream I was standing beside him, holding retractors and looking into the open cavity of the patient's body. The patient was a woman, and the surgeon was pulling her intestines, hand over hand, as if he were reeling a boat in to shore. I was gripping the retractors, but my wrists were starting to fatigue. A strand of hair fell into my face, and I brushed it away with a finger and then held the retractors again, contaminating the sterile field. I knew I had inadvertently placed the patient at risk for infection but was too afraid to say so. Why? Afraid of what? I thought, *This is ridiculous! This operation could fail. This patient could die, and why? Because I'm embarrassed that I made a mistake? Because I don't want this guy to yell at me?* Emboldened, I turned to confront the surgeon, but it was too late. He was gone. I was alone in the room with Lauren, who lay on the operating table, her abdomen agape, holding a needle and thread out to me. 'Go on,' she said. 'Close me, Amazon Brown.'

Waking from the dream, I understood my discomfort with Lauren more deeply. My work with her felt futile. She was *making* me feel futile. Rather than engaging with and exploring that futility, it was simpler, and more fun, to join in the pervasive jokes about zippers and not lending her my pen. Lauren's inexplicable behavior invited this kind of avoidant humor. To look closely at the emotional circumstances that would bring Lauren to swallow a horrifying array of objects demanded a steady gaze fixed firmly on her suffering. Where was the fun in that?

In her riveting book *Swallow: Foreign Bodies, Their Ingestion, Inspiration, and the Curious Doctor Who Extracted Them,* Mary Cappello cites a 1930s article from *Literary Digest* about the intentional ingestion of inedible objects. Its tongue-in-cheek title is 'Iron Rations: Fakirs Swallow Swords, but Amateurs Take Cake Lunching on Hardware'. Cappello describes the article as 'a jaunty piece of journalism that presents the patient, Miss Mabel Wolf, as an amateur when compared to a knife-swallowing Indian magician, but one whose staggering feat far outstrips his. Each sentence is accompanied by a wink and a nudge as if to admit the extremity of her act while keeping all that is disturbing about it at bay. . . . "When she felt depressed," the journalist jokes, "she cheered herself up by indulging in a little nut-and-bolt snack."' In all, Mabel Wolf had swallowed an astonishing array of objects over time

– 1,203 to be exact – an array that included various tacks, screws, bolts, pins, nails, beads, pieces of glass, and safety pins, as well as a coat hanger and the handle of a teacup.

Groaning about Lauren's chronic condition ('a little nut-and-bolt snack') aligned me with my colleagues and the other medical teams. It subconsciously shifted the balance. It became us against her, and there was strength in numbers. If we all knew that Lauren was crazy, then what did it matter what insults she flung my way? If Mabel Wolf was a hysterical depressive, she could be relegated to the circus tent of odd-balls and freaks (and sword swallowers!) and the sane readers of *Literary Digest* could disclaim any similarity between her suffering and their own. On the hospital wards, the jokes about Lauren provided a kind of shared solace. They allowed us to dismiss her as a hopeless case. They quietly identified her as the doctors' adversary rather than a hospitalized patient no less in need of our care than any other.

The increasingly obligatory nature of my visits to Lauren was a sign that more than anything I was ready for her treatment to end. Like my medical and surgical colleagues, I just wanted Lauren to be well enough to leave the hospital. Unfortunately for both Lauren and her doctors, it was clear that being 'well enough' to be discharged from the hospital was a fleeting, ever-changing condition in Lauren's case. Her recurrent, crisis-driven visits to the emergency room and subsequent admissions inflamed a mounting feeling of resentment in her care providers. After Lauren had been discharged and readmitted several times, the medical and surgical teams wanted more than for her to be discharged from their care yet again – they wanted her to be out of their hair for good.

The resentment that Lauren's swallowing bred was mostly directed back toward her. But occasionally the adversarial stances seeped into the ways the medical teams related to one another. One day, outside Lauren's doorway, I ran into the rounding fellow of the GI service.

'Hey,' I said, stopping him in the hall, 'I saw you guys finally got the last of those bulb fragments out, so she's probably pretty close to being able to go from a medical standpoint, huh?'

He turned and looked at me. 'You know,' he began, 'every time she comes in, you guys tell us there's only so much you can do. We pull out whatever life-threatening thing she's decided to eat this time, and as soon as she's medically cleared, you let her go right back home so that she can shove something else down her throat.'

'Well, yeah,' I said. 'I mean, we can't exactly keep her here once she's not in danger anymore.'

'Not *here*,' he replied, gesturing down the hall of the medical floor. 'She should go to Jane 5. And once they won't keep her anymore, she should go to Slater and stay there.' He turned away from me and continued on his rounds, down the hall. Jane 5 was the inpatient psych ward within this medical hospital; the doctors there had admitted and treated Lauren countless times before without significant improvement. They – and we – now felt that constantly admitting her to the psychiatric ward was counterproductive, because it simply extended the duration of her hospitalization and any attention and reinforcement she received from it. Once she was discharged, she had proved to be no less likely to swallow something. And Slater? That was the state mental hospital. The fellow was arguing that Lauren be permanently institutionalized.

I was taken aback by this doctor's suggestion, but in truth his urge to have Lauren put away and prevented from coming back to his service was not too different from my own obligatory visits to her, my avoidance, my wanting her to get just better enough to leave. He made his wish more overt, but, whether or not I was willing to admit it, I shared that desire. I had given up any faith in the possibility of a meaningful recovery for Lauren, one in which she would stabilize and break her cycle of emergent hospitalizations, in which she would find and employ healthy ways of coping with her distress. My anticipation of her discharge did not mean I had some fantasy that she would get better once she left. It was a marker only of the fact that I wouldn't have to be involved in her care any longer.

Sigmund Freud famously identified a number of psychic defense mechanisms – ways in which we unconsciously protect ourselves from being fully aware of thoughts or feelings that are unpleasant to us. Among them is projection, the ego defense in which, rather than acknowledging our own unsettling feelings, we assign them to someone else. Freud's classic example of projection is a spouse (A) who has thoughts of cheating on his partner (B). Instead of dealing with those thoughts, which he finds repugnant, A unconsciously projects his feelings onto his partner, who he becomes convinced may be considering having an affair. By projecting 'his own impulses to faithlessness on to the partner', Freud says, A achieves 'acquittal by conscience' and protects himself from consciously acknowledging his own thoughts of infidelity – a prospect he cannot tolerate.

The famed psychoanalytic thinker Melanie Klein broadened and deepened our understanding of projection. One of her important contributions to object relations theory, the analytic school of thought for which she is best known, is the concept of a defense mechanism called projective identification. Projective identification is related to projection – as a wizardly cousin of sorts. So take again Freud's example of A, the spouse with unfaithful longings. In order to distance himself from his unbearable feelings, A projects them onto B. In projective identification, B, the unsuspecting partner, is initially accused of infidelity without any grounds whatsoever. Over time, however, A's relentless mistrust and jealousy create a distance between the two. B begins finding A irritating and unattractive. Eventually B *does* begin to imagine leaving A for someone who is more alluring and less suspicious.

Hence the wizardry: In projective identification the distressing impulses within one person are displaced – projected – onto another person and thereby *created* within that second person. The dynamic is not magical, of course, but it is powerful, and usually incomprehensible to both members of the dyad because the forces at play are largely unconscious.

I began to understand that projective identification was lying beneath and giving rise to a slew of reactions to Lauren: mine, the medical and surgical teams', the nurses', the hospital's. Her swallowing and her subsequent desperate need for care and attention were always accompanied by her complete disavowal of her deep and persistent need for human responsiveness. Lauren sought care from doctors and nurses – professionals who had chosen to provide care and service to others and who wanted to do so. Then, after seeking our care, Lauren lashed out at us, often by identifying something in us that was actually real. My eyebrows, for example. My height. My privileged place of medical education. *Amazon Brown.* It was this aggression, based in some piece of reality, that hooked us into enacting the script of projective identification. Thus we became angry and abandoning figures who could only harm and disappoint, and in so becoming we enacted and reenacted the traumatic themes of anger and abandonment that had run in swift and ceaseless currents through Lauren's life.

As it does for many people who injure themselves, swallowing dangerous objects somehow brought Lauren a sense of calm when her life felt too chaotic, when she felt vulnerable and attacked. By her swallowing, and the way she treated the doctors obliged to care for her in light of it, Lauren projected her feelings of chaos and inadequacy onto all of us. The results were everywhere, from the swirling mess of staff members angrily dismantling a hospital room in preparation for Lauren's admission to my own self-consciousness, self-doubt, and wish to see her discharged and gone.

We had all internalized Lauren's discomfort and now wanted to push it – and her – away. And therein lies the maladaptive truth of projective identification: It can spark a self-fulfilling prophecy. Fears that infidelity will breach the marital walls *cause* a partner to cheat. Lauren's fears of rejection, abandonment, and aggression lead to behavior that brings about rejection, abandonment, and aggression. Lauren's uncle or sister falls ill, she fights with a neighbor, she swallows rusty scissor blades. We prepare to discharge her from the hospital (yet another form of abandonment and rejection in Lauren's eyes), and she eats chips of wood from the window frame. Soon we all feel angry at Lauren and want her to leave the hospital and never come back.

People who hurt themselves on purpose tend to explain their actions with a shared, if paradoxical, refrain: In situations of extreme stress, self-injury can provide a release. But *how* does this coping mechanism work? How can physical pain relieve psychic pain? How could shedding one's own blood or purging be comforting? How could swallowing a potentially lethal object make a person feel safer?

To attempt to answer these questions – and therefore to be better able to treat Lauren and other patients like her – I needed to examine both what has happened to self-injurers in their lives to lead them to harm themselves and what happens to them when they do.

It is, of course, impossible to make general statements that apply to an entire population. Nonetheless, psychiatrists and their colleagues have identified that trauma, abuse, and neglect can predispose people to self-harm.

Dr Bessel van der Kolk, a psychiatrist and preeminent researcher on the effects of trauma, has repeatedly found that the brain can be structurally and chemically altered by severe trauma. If these changes happen at an early-enough age, the resulting damage may be permanent. Similarly, in their 2000 paper entitled 'Repetitive Self-Injurious

Behavior: A Neuropsychiatric Perspective and Review of Pharmacologic Treatments', Brown University psychiatrists Rendueles Villalba and Colin Harrington write, 'Numerous animal and human studies associate early psychological trauma with subsequent development of repetitive self-injurious behavior.' Villalba and Harrington elaborate on some specific neurological effects of trauma and support van der Kolk's assertion that the brain is changed: 'Overt abuse (especially of a sexual nature), as well as severe neglect, may produce profoundly toxic . . . effects on neuropsychologic development.' They cite nonhuman primate research that found that 'early social isolation frequently leads to repetitive self-injurious behavior' and that primates who were deprived of social contact and support not only hurt themselves but also exhibited changes in both the structure and function of their brains.

These findings hark back to a famous set of experiments with rhesus and macaque monkeys, conducted from the 1950s to the 1970s by Margaret and Harry Harlow. In a series of heartrending studies, the Harlows separated infant monkeys from their mothers, sometimes keeping them in isolation chambers for up to two years. The experiments yielded some of the most durable scientific findings on the psychological and behavioral consequences of social isolation in primates and prompted a radical reexamination of the importance of parent-infant bonding. (They also, unsurprisingly, contributed to the rise of the animal-rights movement.)

The isolated Harlow monkeys were subjected to a variety of environments and stressors, and their responses were dutifully recorded and analyzed. Through their experimentation, the Harlows found that baby monkeys who were isolated differed in many ways from their nonisolated counterparts. 'Total isolation . . . for at least the first six months of life', Harry Harlow writes, 'consistently produces severe deficits in virtually every aspect of social behavior'. Monkeys who had been isolated 'were grossly incompetent' in their social interactions. 'As infants and adolescents', Harlow writes, 'they failed to initiate or reciprocate the play and grooming behaviors characteristic of their peers'. As adults these monkeys did not engage in normal sexual behavior. They showed abnormal levels of aggression. And the females who had been isolated subsequently made terrible mothers, ignoring or behaving violently toward their offspring. Monkeys who had been isolated for six months 'demonstrated limited social recovery' when reintegrated with a primate community. In monkeys who had spent their entire first year of life in total social isolation, no recovery whatsoever was shown. Harry Harlow's discussion of this finding is appropriately grim: 'The effects of six months of total social isolation were so devastating and debilitating that we had assumed initially that twelve months of isolation would not produce any additional decrement. This assumption proved to be false; twelve months of isolation almost obliterated the animals socially.'

Many of the baby monkeys who were separated from their mothers exhibited self-injurious behavior when afraid. Some banged their heads against their cages. Others hit themselves. Still others bit their own extremities, sometimes to the point of near amputation. As these monkeys were subjected to increasingly stressful situations and stimuli, some hurt themselves so badly that they had to be euthanized. The responses the primates had to the self-harm were particularly striking in that they mirrored the sequence of emotions described by humans who intentionally inflict injury upon themselves: When the monkeys began hurting themselves, they were agitated and visibly distressed. As their self-injury progressed, they became calmer and calmer.

So what is it about self-mutilation that has the power to produce calm in a certain cohort of human and nonhuman primates alike?

From a scientific standpoint, self-injurious behavior is difficult to study. The ethics of scientific research prevent studies from being conducted in which human subjects are knowingly harmed, and rightly so. However, this means that we cannot, for example, observe cutters as they are cutting themselves in order to assess the physiological and psychological responses their actions evoke. Instead researchers must rely on patients' self-reporting – a notoriously inexact source of data – or devise experiments that attempt to replicate the effects of cutting without in fact causing harm.

In 1995 the *Journal of Abnormal Psychology* published a paper by Janet Haines and her colleagues entitled 'The Psychophysiology of Self-Mutilation', which aimed to do precisely that. In the paper, Haines lists the reported factors that give rise to the negative emotions that most commonly prompt self-injury as 'interpersonal conflict, rejection, separation, or abandonment', which may be 'threatened, real, or imagined'. Indeed, nearly all of Lauren's admissions cited predisposing events that could be interpreted through this lens. A terminally ill uncle or a sister's hepatitis diagnosis could signal pending abandonment via illness or death. A fight with a neighbor raised the specter of both interpersonal conflict and personal rejection. Similarly, when Lauren's doctors and nurses grew frustrated by her behavior and impatient with her care, she would perceive this as yet another rejection. In the self-fulfilling prophecy of projective identification, her own actions poured fuel on the fire of her worst fears.

Haines describes a generalized sequence of events that typically occur before, during, and after self-injury. This sequence has been repeatedly described by self-injurers and their clinicians, and it begins with the rise of negative emotions. As the emotions swell, they reach a point where the self-injurer can no longer tolerate the intensity of the feelings. It is at this point that a phenomenon called dissociation is thought to occur. Haines writes that as the negative feelings become increasingly intolerable, 'many self-mutilators report feeling numb, withdrawn, and unreal' and begin to engage in the act of harming themselves. As the wound is inflicted, it typically does not cause pain until 'minutes, hours, or even days after the injury', regardless of its severity. Haines postulates that this anesthesia is likely a physiological one, 'mediated by an increase in endogenous opiates . . . caused by the extreme stress reaction prior to cutting'. In other words, according to her theory, the body may release its own morphinelike substances twice: first in response to the stress and then in response to the injury. Not only would this double response mute pain, it also could contribute to the addictive properties of self-injury, reinforcing the impulse to turn to self-harm in moments of distress.

Haines wanted to explore exactly what happens in the body and mind during episodes of self-injury. In order to do this, she gathered groups of 'mutilators' and 'nonmutilators' and read them personalized scripts of various events they had experienced and described, including one event, such as an argument with a significant other, that was meant to evoke a degree of psychic distress. Then both groups were read a script that guided them through images of self-harm. Various physiological measurements associated with tension, such as pulse and respiratory rate, were taken throughout the experiments. The results showed that the subjects with a history of self-injurious behavior became calmer – both by their own self-assessment and by the measured bodily responses – during the self-mutilation imagery. Essentially, the mere act of imagining they were hurting themselves calmed the 'mutilators' down. No such results were evoked from the 'nonmutilator' subject group.

Months after I encountered Lauren, I treated a woman who, in the context of her husband's moving out, had cut her wrists with a razor blade. 'I felt so empty, so separate from myself, I didn't even really notice I was doing it,' she recounted to me, her thin forearms wrapped in gauze. 'Or I noticed, but it was more like I was watching it happen from above, not participating in it. At some point I saw something glistening white, and that kind of snapped me out of it. I remember thinking, "What are those white lines interrupting the red?" and then I realized they were my tendons, and then I saw how much blood was all around me. *That's* the only time I got scared. Not because it hurt – it didn't, it hadn't – but because I suddenly realized that I was going to have to go to the hospital.' She paused. 'I knew that my sister would be really upset. I guess I only freaked out because I realized what a mess I had made and how badly I had screwed up.'

This numbness and disconnection that my patient described help elucidate the phenomenon of dissociation. The self becomes an outsider who observes the body from afar, who does not participate in its actions and does not feel its feelings, be they emotional or physical. *Foreign body.*

To a certain degree, dissociation can be a normal part of our everyday lives. I may feed the dog, brush my teeth, empty the dishwasher, yet on any given day have no recollection of the steps I took in the process of each of these mundane, everyday occurrences. I had the attention to complete these tasks but not the conscious awareness of doing so. 'Highway hypnosis' is another common form of dissociation in which people may drive for long distances without clear recollections of shifting gears or maneuvering in traffic, without an awareness of having navigated turns and off-ramps on their way to their destination.

Trauma is understood to cause a spectrum of more serious dissociative symptoms. A mild form of dissociation may occur in the midst of grief when, after the death of a loved one, we feel as if we are floating above ourselves or wading through a thick emotional fog, unable to connect with others or respond to our lives in the ways we normally do. After the September 11 attacks, hordes of New York City residents reported uncharacteristic feelings of detachment and disconnectedness. Scientific research has linked high levels of dissociative symptoms to the aftermaths of war, of earthquakes, of torture, of firestorms. Studies have demonstrated that people are far more likely to embody a dissociative state after they have witnessed an execution. The psychiatrist Glen Gabbard, a renowned psychoanalytic scholar, explains these occurrences succinctly. 'Dissociation', he writes, 'allows individuals to retain an illusion of psychological control when they experience a sense of helplessness and loss of control over their bodies'. The type of dissociation that permits self-harm, however, is obviously less benign than that which results from inattention, or even from grief.

Not all people who endure trauma – or even all those who exhibit dissociative symptoms in its wake – engage in self-injurious behavior. In her illuminating 1998 book on self-injury, *A Bright Red Scream,* the journalist Marilee Strong turns to attachment theory to explain why this is so. Attachment theory postulates that a child's ability to develop into a psychically healthy individual is largely dependent upon whether there has been a stable emotional bond between the child and an adult who cares for him. A secure attachment bond assures the child that he is safe and that he will survive. Strong writes, 'Research has confirmed that a single secure attachment bond is the most powerful protection against traumatization. Emotional attachment makes a child feel connected and supported, not alone and helpless. . . . Abused and neglected children never learn from their parents how to soothe themselves and cannot trust others to help them do so. So they may turn to cutting and other forms of self-injury as a means of self-soothing and reestablishing, at least temporarily, biological and psychological equilibrium.' Strong goes on to quote the psychologist David Frankel. 'Usually kids internalize a sense of a parent they can call up from inside themselves for comfort in times of distress', says Frankel. 'These kids don't have that – or what they call up is a Mom who wishes they were dead and a Dad who wants to sleep with them.'

Dr Diana Lidofsky, a psychologist and the director of psychotherapy training at Brown, elaborates upon Frankel's assertion. Abusive parents who are intentionally malevolent certainly exist and may give rise to children who harm themselves, she agrees. Still, she believes that the parental failures that predispose a child to self-injurious behavior are more commonly based in deep neglect. Lidofsky characterizes this neglect as 'chronic and toxic misattunement'. These parents, she asserts, may not physically or sexually abuse their children but may instead be 'catastrophically absent, inadequate, and disturbed'.

In people who deliberately hurt themselves, dissociation has often taken root as a coping mechanism in the midst of trauma. When a child is beaten or neglected or sexually abused, she may dissociate in order to distance herself from the experience. If she cannot physically get away from her abuse or neglect, she finds psychic ways to do so. If a person has to dissociate frequently, she may eventually shift into a state in which she perpetually feels disconnected and numb.

Self-injury, then, with its flood of sensation, pierces this feeling of unreality and deadness. A razor blade splits flesh, and bright red blood pours forth and stains everything in its path. The hot metal rim of a lighter presses into skin, and smoke issues forth, carrying with it a jarring, searing smell of burn. Hair is torn from the scalp, tangling fingers in knotted tresses. A cold scissor blade slides down Lauren's throat, and it is gripped and held by esophagus, sphincter, stomach; an ache persists, locatable, its cause known.

One day during Lauren's hospitalization, I realized I didn't know anything about her childhood or her family, and I decided to ask her. She was so furious with me that she would not even speak. Though she was choosing not to engage in her treatment, I didn't want to do the same. So I returned to Lauren's lengthy charts, in which I had first found a record of all she had ingested and all the ways in which the objects had been removed. Lauren was such a familiar patient to everyone else who worked in the hospital that I had picked up her care in the present moment, as if her history were as well known to me as it was to the doctors who had cared for her so many times before. I went back to Lauren's earliest records to treat her like a brand-new patient, in the hope that I could find something we were all overlooking that could actually *help* her. I wanted to let go of all the behavioral plans and baggage that accompanied Lauren the minute she arrived in the

ER; I wanted to let go of my own frustration and release the feelings of ineptitude she gave rise to in me.

The psychiatric and medical and surgical notes of Lauren's current admission no longer contained the detailed descriptions that might have characterized a first, second, or even third hospitalization. Instead the notes were full of shorthand phrases that summarized her years of treatment as a chronic patient. She was a 'well-known' patient with a 'long history of intentional ingestions'. A patient who had 'failed multiple medication trials', for whom an established care plan was immediately put in place. I had come to know her this way, as a prepackaged, well-known patient with a huge reputation. A chronic patient. A patient who had consistently failed to be cured.

I laboriously paged through Lauren's charts. I did not come away with a treatment plan I hoped would save her. Yet I did find, back in her earliest admissions, a deeper understanding of her past.

Lauren's father was murdered when she was a baby. She never knew her mother for reasons that are not clear. Her aunt, who took her in after her father died, was a heroin addict and died from an accidental overdose when Lauren was six. From that time on, Lauren lived in a series of group homes and foster homes. She used drugs and sometimes stole or prostituted herself to get them. Her psychiatric admissions started when she was in elementary school and never stopped. She had given birth to two children, both of whom were immediately taken into protective custody and never returned to her. They would have now been eleven and six, born when Lauren was fourteen and nineteen, respectively.

I didn't have to know about rhesus monkeys in isolation or the intricacies of attachment theory to imagine that a person with Lauren's history might be acutely sensitive to abandonment. Whether or not trauma had brought about physical changes in her brain that I could not see, I could believe that she'd had experiences during which it was better to be numb, distant, floating.

Even if we understand why Lauren and others may chronically hurt themselves and why the behavior is helpful to them (if only partially and temporarily so), the challenges of how to treat these patients within our current health-care system do not fade.

As doctors' reactions to Lauren and her chronic need for medical and surgical intervention illustrated, these patients bring up ethical quandaries and complicated emotional reactions for the doctors involved in their care.

One such example was a mentally ill twenty-year-old man who was winter camping with his family when he heard the voice of Jesus instructing him to cut off his hand with the hatchet he was using to chop wood. Believing it to be a holy command, he did so and returned to the campsite. His distraught parents frantically searched for the amputated hand. When they found it, they packed it in snow and ice and drove the young man, and his severed hand, to the hospital.

Hours passed before the young man was seen by hand surgeons, and when he was, the team expressed concern that too much time had gone by and that as a result the surgery would not be successful. In their decision making, they also discussed with the family their concerns about how the patient's mental health would affect the likelihood of surgical success. He would need to be lucid enough to follow a detailed regimen of postoperative care, critical for proper healing. The doctors feared that the man's mental state rendered him likely to jeopardize the fragile reattachment. Any attempt at rejoining the hand to the wrist would be a procedure of at least twenty-two hours in length. If, at worst, he continued to feel compelled to remove his hand or if, at least, he was not well enough to scrupulously care for it once it was reattached, the extraordinary effort and resources required for such an operation would have been wasted. In the end the hand surgeons decided not to operate, citing the passage of too much time since the accident.

The distraught family frantically drove to another hospital for a second opinion, where they were told that their arrival at the first hospital had in fact been within the window of timing where such a procedure would have been possible but that they were now beyond it. The family sought legal redress against the surgeons at the first hospital, believing that the true impetus for refusing care had been a form of discrimination, that their son had been denied appropriate care because he was mentally ill.

It may well have been that the rationale the surgeons expressed – that too much time had passed for the operation to have been a success – was true. However, since the second surgical team disagreed, it is worth considering the ethical issues at play: the dilemma raised as to whether or not this patient was an appropriate surgical candidate, irrespective of time. It is not difficult to imagine that had the patient been psychiatrically well and had severed his hand in an accident rather than on purpose, the surgical team might even have been willing to attempt the procedure at the outermost cusp of the appropriate time frame, given the grave repercussions of the loss of such a vital body part.

So what was the right thing to do for this young man in this scenario? Does every patient deserve a chance at the repair of a permanent and grievous injury – no matter how complicated or expensive – even if there is a substantial risk that the restorative effort will be unsuccessful or, worse, *undone*? When psychiatric illness also requires medical or surgical care, which takes precedence: the severity of the body's afflictions or the severity of those of the mind? Can the presence of one type of illness preclude receiving treatment for the other? If the surgeons should be obliged to attempt to reconnect this patient's hand, would they also be obliged to operate if he cut it off a second time or intentionally interfered with its healing? What criteria would have to be met in order for it to be ethical for a doctor to refuse to intervene?

A patient like this one differs from Lauren in significant ways: He is psychotic, whereas she is seen to be more 'in control' of her thoughts and actions; therefore, her self-injury is seen as more volitional. Cutting off a hand with a hatchet is a dramatic onetime act, shocking and tragic, with severe long-term consequences. Lauren's chronic ingestions, which thus far have been reversible and nonlethal, are seen as more annoyance than catastrophe. Nonetheless, there are many similarities between the two patients: Both have self-inflicted wounds that will have fatal or life-altering consequences if not treated; both are likely – though not guaranteed – to repeat the behavior that caused the injury in the first place. Why, then, is Lauren consistently admitted and treated (even with her own personal treatment protocol) when for the young man camping in winter the decision was not so straightforward?

The answer may lie in the relative complexity of the treatments. Although endoscopy, too, is a medical procedure, it is unquestionably less involved, less time-consuming, and less expensive than limb-reattachment surgery would be. However, given the fact that Lauren has had dozens of procedures and in all likelihood will have more in her future, the cumulative resources required may well exceed those of a onetime surgery, even one as complicated as reattaching a hand.

I wonder if the difference lies instead in reaction versus prevention, in the risks in medicine associated with omission versus those associated with commission. When the young man came in with his hand packed in ice, the worst had already happened. His hand was severed; any action taken by doctors would be an attempt to remediate the situation. The doctors could certainly choose to undertake the heroic task of reattachment, but they needed to weigh the costs and perils against the potential benefit. Whether the risk they counted most heavily was the time that had elapsed since the accident or the patient's psychosis, in the end they believed that the chance of a good outcome was not substantial enough to overcome the odds of failure.

Lauren's actions also had already taken place by the time she reached the hospital, but, in contrast to the young man's amputation, the worst possible damage for Lauren had not yet occurred. With Lauren, doctors were consistently in a position where their intervention could *prevent* disaster. By sending her to endoscopy and removing the objects she ingested, they averted the perforation of her gastrointestinal tract. If they opted not to treat her, their inaction could be linked to her catastrophe.

This critical difference speaks to the very nature of the distinction between major and superficial/moderate self-harm. For the young winter camper, the key to his recovery would lie in the treatment of his psychosis. Although the loss of his hand is an irrevocable tragedy, our current psychiatric system of care is not bad at treating auditory command hallucinations. In all likelihood, with intensive psychiatric treatment, a safe and structured environment, and antipsychotic medications, we would eventually be able to stop him from believing that Jesus wanted him to maim himself (though almost certainly not within the time frame of any surgical repair and postoperative care that could have occurred). With ongoing treatment, chances are that he might go years, decades, even his whole life without ever trying to hurt himself again.

Those odds are far less likely for Lauren. The crisis and mandatory call to action brought about by her repetitive swallowing are both a symptom of her illness and its fuel. Whatever isolation or trauma may have bred this incomprehensible means of relieving her distress, that gaping hole is now filled with the constant, emergent attention of medical and surgical teams, psychiatric consultants, security guards, even hospital administrators. We attend to her urgent needs – we ethically cannot refuse to do so. But in attending to them, we reinforce her understanding that she can glean care from her ingestions; we strengthen the positive feedback loop of her repetitive self-injury.

As her psychiatric consultant, I felt that my limited time with her underscored the problem with this form of treatment. Because Lauren was primarily a medical or surgical patient, my role with her was limited by definition. I was not primarily responsible for her treatment; my job was only to provide recommendations for the psychiatric component of her care: How could we keep Lauren safe in the hospital? How could we try to keep attention to her at a minimum while providing appropriate medical, surgical, and psychiatric care? The *real* work of her treatment needed to be done on an outpatient basis, when she wasn't in crisis, when someone would have enough time to treat her with psychotherapy that would address both this cycle and the psychic wounds out of which it sprang.

But this treatment plan for her discharge was not a completely honest one. Lauren was never 'not in crisis'. She had been admitted to the hospital twenty-three times in the last four years. She had never maintained any kind of a long-term outpatient therapeutic relationship. Like it or not, realistic or not, we *were* her primary-care physicians.

During each of my subsequent visits with Lauren, she was dismissive of me, alternating between loud, monosyllabic, often vulgar responses and complete silence. I regained my footing in our clinical encounters, and I stopped taking her vitriol personally. In fact, I'm not at all sure that there wasn't something appropriate about her response. I was purporting to be there to help her. I would leave the room and write a long note with some minor changes to her psychiatric medications and a set of standard recommendations for outpatient care, knowing that the first was unlikely to help and the second was unlikely to happen. I did it in good faith. They were the 'right' recommendations. But I was part of the only treatment plan a crisis-based hospital could muster. I was approaching the patient with a 'focus on disease management, not cure'. Like the lightbulbs, the knife blades, and the curtain rods, I was at best a temporary easement, a learned pattern that might diminish distress in the short term but constantly needed to be repeated and never had any kind of lasting effect.

One night after seeing Lauren, I returned home to find my children getting ready for bed, all warm with shampooed hair and toothpaste drips down their fleece pajama tops. When they saw me setting down my bag and unclipping my pager from my waistband, they raced toward me, tumbling over each other. They had, all day, been listening to the song in *Mary Poppins* in which Jane and Michael Banks have written the description of their ideal nanny, and they wanted to perform it for me.

'Be an audience, Mama!' my two-year-old boy shouted, as instructed by his older sister, though he had no concept of what an audience might be. I flopped onto the couch to watch as they crooned and giggled to an imaginary nanny, 'Love us as a son and daughter. / And never smell of barley water!' As their song gave rise to an improvised dance and they began to march around the living room, I found my mind shifting back to Lauren. It felt out of place to be thinking of her here, with her dark stares and her prickly anger, but I could not shake the feeling that I was doing her a grave disservice. Later that evening, with the kids packed off to bed, Deborah and I sat at our dining-room table, plates cleared, a half-empty bottle of wine between us. I explained to her how I was feeling.

'The system is broken,' I told her. She was unconvinced.

'That may be,' she said. 'But how can you discharge her with a plan that you know isn't going to help her? That you know isn't going to work?'

'It's more complicated than that,' I bristled, and Deborah quieted, looking down. I felt anger swell up inside me, and I knew it was because she was right.

The next day at the hospital, as I prepared for Lauren's imminent discharge, I threw myself into creating an aftercare plan for her that would be more than a formality, one that actually had a chance of helping her break this cycle of admission after admission. Without insurance or money to self-pay for her treatment, Lauren did not have the option of seeing a private psychiatrist or psychotherapist. If she did, she might have been seen by a therapist every week for an hour and a psychiatrist once or twice a month. Instead Lauren was treated by an overextended, publicly funded mental-health center where she was scheduled to see a psychiatrist for twenty minutes four times a year. Of course, in one of the ironies that are all too common in a country with health-care discrepancies, a single hospital admission for Lauren – paid by the taxpayer-funded state medical-assistance program – cost more than a year of private outpatient care would.

I called the psychiatrist at the mental-health center to whom Lauren was assigned and learned from him that one of the center's only other psychiatrists had recently quit. With an ever-increasing caseload and an ever-shrinking budget, he said, there was no chance of her being seen more frequently. I had him transfer me to Lauren's case manager to inquire if she could at least be seen by him more regularly. Lauren didn't keep her appointments, the case manager told me. True, he said, she had no car and lived miles outside the bus route. 'Look . . .' He paused. 'There's only so much I can do. I can't help her if she doesn't come in.' I asked about the center's mobile treatment team that goes to patients' homes, takes them their medications, drives them to their appointments. 'I guess it's possible,' the case manager said. 'She'd have to be evaluated by them. Let me check the book.' I waited on hold for several minutes. I was eventually disconnected. I called back. 'Oh, hey,' the case manager said. 'Yeah, I can book her for an appointment for a mobile treatment team eval. Our first available opening is June twenty-third.' It was now February.

I headed to Lauren's room. She had been fully cleared by the medical team, and they were awaiting our confirmation that she was safe to leave the hospital. I had her outpatient-care plan in my hands, and it included Lauren's appointment to be seen by the mobile treatment team, though a long four months away. And much of the plan had a chance only if she diligently followed it and if the realities of her poverty and her limited sources of emotional support didn't intrude, as they would, as they always had. I knocked on her door, and as I stood waiting for her to respond, I still felt I had done almost nothing for this patient.

'Who is it?' Lauren finally yelled.

'Amazon Brown,' I answered.

In response I heard a sound I had never heard from her: a chuckle of laughter. Then, 'Come in.'

As I entered, I thought of something a beloved supervisor said to me during my training, about working with difficult patients. 'Sometimes holding all the blackness they feel is the only thing you can do. That's not nothing. And sometimes it is enough.'

'Hey,' I said. 'I understand they're ready to let you go. How do you feel about that?'

'Oh, Jesus, with the "How do you feel?" shit again,' she moaned, although this time there was a current of nervousness beneath her tone. 'I hate this place! I've been wanting to get the fuck out of here for days.'

I handed her the number I had for her case manager. 'So, Lauren,' I began, 'if you can bring yourself to do it, next time you're upset and you feel the urge to swallow something, you might try calling first.'

'Why would I do a stupid thing like that?' she asked.

'Well,' I said, 'maybe they could help.'

She scoffed.

'And more than anything, Lauren, I'm afraid that one of these times you're going to swallow something and it's not going to go this way. I mean, I'm afraid you could swallow something and then you could die.'

She rolled her eyes. 'Like that'd be so bad.'

'I think it would be,' I said softly. 'I think it would be terrible.' She looked up at me, and for a minute I thought maybe she heard me.

'Yeah, well,' Lauren said, 'you'd be the only one.'

I held out my hand to her to shake, and she took it. 'Take care of yourself,' I said.

To which she responded, 'When can I get my stuff and get out of here?'

That evening I wrote in my consult note that I believed Lauren was safe for discharge. I didn't feel the relief I thought I would at her impending departure. I mostly felt sad. Not because I would be sorry to have her off my service but because I felt that the treatment she'd received this time – like so many other times in the past and surely more to come – was just a gesture, a Band-Aid on a gaping wound.

I headed down the hospital staircase to gather my coat and bag from the psychiatry office. I checked my pager one last time, and when I raised my eyes from its numbered screen, they fixed on the stairwell's wall ahead of me: the poster, the horses. *Whose woods these are I think I know. / His house is in the village, though; / He will not see me stopping here / To watch his woods fill up with snow.*

When I push open the hospital doors to walk through the many parking lots to my car, sharp, frigid air enters my lungs and makes me gasp. I cough a little. Inhale deeply. The cold air like a stab. My exhalation leaves moisture on my face that freezes instantly and makes my cheeks hurt as I walk. I am moving quickly, hurrying to the car, to home. Each step of my dress shoe on the cold, hard pavement makes my foot ache. It reminds me of the ringing jolt of pain in my hands I'd feel in Little League when I'd hit a baseball hard on a cold day and the bat would send the force straight to my palms. I get it – we all must – how pain can quicken the heart and then, with each pulse's beat, send a message to the mind. *A-live. A-live. A-live.*

Months later – it is May – I am standing thigh-deep in the northern Michigan lake of my childhood. It's a holy place to me, one to which I return year after year. Only a month ago, the lake was frozen stiff, and it will be a good month yet before anyone else in my family will venture into the water. I walk out farther still. The water laps the borders of my swimsuit. I cannot feel my feet. My children are shouting with glee on the dock, egged on by Deborah, who laughs and cheers, 'Look at Mama! Look at her in the cold water!' I give a broad wave, take a deep breath in, and then I dive. It is so cold that my whole self hurts. Icicles to my scalp, my eyes. I leap up immediately, spin, and shriek at my children, who jump up and down and happily shriek back. Deborah yells something triumphant I cannot decipher. I wrap my arms around myself and run – splashing frigid droplets in a wide spray around me – toward the dock, their happy voices. I cannot believe this joy, this fullness of my life.

CHAPTER TWO

Fifty-Thousand-Dollar Skin

*And if thy right hand offend thee, cut it off, and cast it from thee:
for it is profitable for thee that one of thy members should perish,
and not that thy whole body should be cast into hell.*

— Matthew 5:30

Late in my residency training, I had an outpatient practice in which I saw patients longitudinally over the course of a year. It was there that I first met thirty-four-year-old Eddie. When Eddie came to see me, he had just moved to Rhode Island from Utah. As a result, several months had passed since he had last seen his previous psychiatrist, and his antidepressant prescription had run out weeks earlier. With the gap in medication, Eddie's always-troubling symptoms had worsened dramatically.

'My skin is awful,' he said in a hushed tone filled with sad urgency. 'And now, to top it off, do you see how my hair is thinning all across the back of my head here?' I didn't. Eddie's skin looked totally normal to me, and I could not see the faintest trace of thinning hair in the area of his scalp toward which he gestured. No one would look at Eddie and think of him either as balding or as having unattractive skin. Still, I neither argued with Eddie nor reassured him – I knew from reading his chart that whether or not I agreed with his self-perceptions was immaterial.

'I've saved up all summer for a treatment,' he continued, referring to his work in a seasonal family restaurant. 'My dermatologist told me about this new laser that goes at the acne scarring from underneath, so I'm hopeful maybe that will help, since nothing else has.' I did not share Eddie's hope for improvement. Since the time he was eighteen, convinced that he had horrific acne scarring that made him repulsive to look at, Eddie had undergone dermatologic procedures as often as he could afford them: painful dermabrasion in which a high-speed rotary instrument with an abrasive wheel was used to remove the outer layers of his skin, repeated laser treatments, silicone injections, 'desiccation' procedures in which supposedly scarred areas of his skin were burned, even a face lift in his late twenties.

Eddie conservatively estimated the number of procedures he had undergone at twenty-five. He guessed he had probably spent close to fifty thousand dollars in an attempt to 'repair' his skin. At his worst, unable to afford a medical procedure and still convinced that his acne scarring was horribly disfiguring, Eddie scoured his face with sandpaper in an attempt to smooth its surface.

Now that the pace of summer work was slowing, Eddie had days when he spent hours at home, constantly in front of the mirror. 'Some mornings I wake up and think my skin actually looks okay,' he explained, 'and then I go back to the mirror to check after breakfast, and the sun is shining in the window and I can see how disgusting the scars are.

'Everyone I know hopes for sunny days,' he went on, 'but whenever I see the clear sky, I know it will only highlight how messed up my face is.' When I asked Eddie how much time he was spending in front of the mirror, he paused to calculate. 'Yesterday? Maybe five hours. The day before?' He paused again to think. 'Maybe eight.'

Eddie's thoughts about his skin and hair not only consumed his mind, they also interfered with the most basic aspects of his life. His girlfriend of many years had left him, fed up with the ways in which his preoccupations with his appearance affected their lives. In addition to the hours Eddie spent each day in front of the mirror, he also canceled plans to go out at the last minute, fearful that he was so hideous-looking that strangers would ridicule him on the street or that in a different light his new girlfriend would finally see him realistically and break up with him on the spot. He would ask her – sometimes hundreds of times a day – how his skin and hair looked. No matter how reassuring her comments were, he remained unconvinced that he was anything other than grotesquely disfigured.

To make matters worse, Eddie was ashamed of his inability to change either his outlook or his behavior. 'Some people think I'm really vain,' he said softly. 'But people who are vain think they are beautiful and *like* to look at themselves.' He paused. 'I hate looking in the mirror, but I have to try to fix how horrible I look.'

Though Eddie's symptoms sound remarkable, the fact is that in terms of the demographics of mental illness his affliction is as common as schizophrenia, anorexia, or bipolar disorder, plaguing one out of every fifty to a hundred people. Descriptions of the disorder can be found even in centuries-old case reports with a range of evocative names, like 'imagined ugliness' and 'dysmorphophobia', but the crux of the symptoms is the same: a preoccupation with an imagined defect in one's appearance or excessive concern about a slight physical anomaly. Today we call this illness body dysmorphic disorder (BDD).

Descriptions of patients who would today be diagnosed with BDD periodically surface in the psychiatric literature of the nineteenth and twentieth centuries. *The Oxford English Dictionary* dates the word 'dysmorphophobia' (from the Greek *dysmorpho-*, meaning 'misshapen or deformed', and *-phobia,* meaning 'fear') to 1891. The first use of the term is attributed to the Italian psychiatrist Enrico Morselli, who gave his article the enticing title 'Dysmorphophobia and Taphephobia'. The fear of being deformed, alongside the fear of being buried alive. The triumphant subtitle of Morselli's article reads like an exploration of the new world: 'Two Hitherto Undescribed Forms of Insanity with Fixed Ideas'. Morselli writes, 'The dysmorphophobic, indeed, is a veritably unhappy individual, who in the midst of his daily affairs, in conversations, while reading, at table, in fact anywhere and at any hour of the day, is suddenly overcome by the fear of some deformity that might have developed in his body without his noticing it.'

Like Bethlem's Charles Harold Wrigley in 1890, the patients whom Morselli describes are indistinguishable from those I see more than a century later. He writes that the dysmorphophobe 'fears having or developing a compressed, flattened forehead, a ridiculous nose, crooked legs, etc., so that he constantly peers in the mirror, feels his forehead, measures the length of his nose, examines the tiniest defects in his skin, or measures the proportions of his trunk and the straightness of his limbs, and only after a certain period of time, having convinced himself that this has not happened, is able to free himself from the state of pain and anguish the attack put him in. But should no mirror be at hand, or should he be prevented from quieting his doubts in some way or other by means of some mechanism or movements of the most outlandish kinds, . . . the attack does not end very quickly, but may reach a very painful intensity, even to the point of weeping and desperation.'

Indeed, patients with BDD, both current and historical, are frequently in true agony, their lives dominated by their constant symptoms. They may check the body part in question hundreds of times a day, smoothing their hair, touching or sizing up whatever it is they believe to be errant.

Eddie's case is not atypical among patients who live with BDD, in that he spends hours looking closely at – and being tormented by – his perceived flaws and going to great lengths in an attempt to correct them. Still, the details of patients' suffering can vary dramatically, even within a single diagnosis. Another of my patients routinely digs into the pores of her face with needles. A third has spent tens of thousands of dollars on multiple elaborate cosmetic dental surgeries. She remains convinced that her teeth are 'disgusting' and has gone to numerous dentists in an attempt to find one who will 'just pull' all of them 'and start over'.

Patients with BDD may endlessly compare themselves to others. One patient told me that she lost her job as a bank teller because she would watch each customer walk away and then have to go into the bathroom to look in the mirror to attempt to assess whether her thighs were bigger or smaller than those of the customer she had helped.

Stricken with the belief that they will be seen as hideous by others, people suffering from BDD will isolate themselves to varying degrees. Many will decline social invitations. Many will be hours late to events because they are stuck rewashing and styling their hair over and over or are unable to tear themselves away from the mirror, examining their perceived deficits. Some miss the weddings of siblings, of best friends. A few refuse to leave their homes at all, trapped by their obsessive thoughts, their fear of others' judgments, and their own self-hatred.

These patients view their flaws as horrific and thus impossible for others not to see and shrink from. In fact, the traits about which they obsess are hardly noticeable, if they are noticeable at all. The patients may even focus on an imperceptible flaw – crooked toes, for instance – while feeling no discomfort at all about traits we might imagine *could* give rise to insecurity, such as baldness or weight gain. In many cases the actions taken in an attempt to *fix* the problem are what draw negative attention to the person's appearance – as when Eddie's dermatologic procedures would leave his skin raw or his face bruised, when patients' minuscule blemishes were picked and poked until they transformed into large and angry sores, when one patient drenched her head with tonics that left her hair coated in an oily sheen, when another combed his hair so compulsively that it caused his scalp to bleed.

In my residency practice, I treated a number of patients with BDD and was incredibly fortunate to be supervised in weekly meetings by Dr Katharine Phillips, the world's preeminent expert on the disease. Dr Phillips speaks openly about the drastic measures that have been taken by her own patients in an attempt to camouflage or rid themselves of their perceived flaws. One patient would not leave her home because she believed she had a hair mask on her face, like a gorilla. Another patient wore a curtain of bangs obscuring her face, down to her chin, in order to hide what she felt was a disfigured nose. The patient had had three rhinoplasties – nose jobs – at the Mayo Clinic, one of the world's most renowned medical centers, and had a nose that most objective bystanders would classify as perfect. She eventually did cut her bangs, only to wear a face mask over her nose and mouth for three years. Instead of functioning as camouflage, these tactics brought even more public attention to her appearance than her flawless nose would ever have done, paradoxically increasing her anxiety further. Eventually her symptoms improved, but only when she engaged fully in a combined treatment program of psychotherapy and psychiatric medications.

The illness sounds fantastically odd, but the consequences can be grave. Patients with BDD often unintentionally harm themselves, sometimes severely. Dr Phillips describes a woman who picked so deeply at a blemish on her neck that her tweezers reached all the way down to the fragile sheath surrounding her carotid artery. She tells of a man who performed self-surgery to try to implant the cartilage he had whittled down from a chicken carcass into his own 'malformed' nose. Her patients have superglued ears they perceive to stick out too far. They have used staple guns to perform home face lifts. A woman allowed her nose to sunburn and peel, sunburn and peel, over and over again in the hope that the constant peeling would somehow make her nose smaller. A man cut off fingers on one hand that he perceived to be too long. A young woman felt that her nipples were 'grotesque' and carved them from her chest.

The greatest danger, however, to Eddie and others who suffer from BDD is that they are at a significantly increased risk of suicide. Eighty percent of patients with BDD will have death wishes or thoughts of killing themselves. Twenty-five percent will try to end their own lives. The rate of completed suicides among BDD patients is about thirty-one times that of the general population.

I treated Eddie for a year. Each time I saw him, I asked whether he had thoughts of killing himself. Each time he said no, but I didn't find his rationale reassuring. 'I want to be dead, yeah,' he'd say with his characteristic candor, 'but I don't know whether I could bring myself to do it. I think I'd be too scared to carry it through. If someone with a gun asked for my wallet, though . . .' And here he paused until I gestured for him to continue. 'I'd say, "Shoot. Go right ahead."'

Eddie's passive suicidality – wishing he were dead but not actively planning to kill himself – arose directly from his unrelenting torment. Though tragic, and a call for real intervention, Eddie's thought process nevertheless contained a misguided logic. So overcome by hopelessness and so miserable, he felt that only death would bring him relief. As his doctor, I could understand how he had come to that place of desperation, but I could also help to foster hope. I reminded him that in the past, with antidepressants and psychotherapy, he had felt better and had been glad to be alive. We could – and would – try to get him back to that place.

In addition to the increased risk of suicide, BDD symptoms can cause such profound psychic distress that people will endure unimaginable physical pain in an attempt to alleviate their bodily concerns. Dr Phillips treated a man who, when fifteen surgeons refused to perform elaborate cosmetic procedures on his face, planned an automobile accident in which he could 'destroy' his face and force doctors to reconstruct it. The plan had an additional benefit: Even if he had found a doctor willing to conduct the elective procedures, his insurance wouldn't have covered them, as they would have been deemed cosmetic, and he would not have been able to afford to pay for them. An accident, he reasoned, would certainly be covered by insurance.

Another of Dr Phillips's patients, a woman she calls Julie, became absolutely obsessed with the possibility of harming her nose. Twenty years prior to being seen by Dr Phillips, Julie had had minor surgery on her nose to 'remove a small bump'. 'After surgery', Phillips writes in her book on BDD, *The Broken Mirror,* 'the surgeon commented, "I worked really hard on your nose, so take care of it and don't damage it." Julie took this to mean that her nose was fragile, and it triggered her obsession.'

In the years that followed, Julie constantly went to her surgeon's office – sometimes twice a week, sometimes waiting two hours to be seen – seeking reassurance that she had not inadvertently, unknowingly, broken her nose. Julie told Dr Phillips that she had been unable to work and unable to keep her house in order: 'I'm so focused on my nose that I can't think of anything else.' This had not been the first time that her fears had become so all-encompassing. Julie told Dr Phillips that her preoccupation was 'a huge problem in my marriage, too. My first husband left me because of it. I drove him nuts! I asked him all day long about my nose and whether I'd damaged it, and I'd have him hold magnifying glasses and special lights to check it for damage.' Julie's fear that her nose might be harmed dwarfed her fear and experience of actual physical pain. Dr Phillips writes, 'During childbirth, Julie was so petrified that her nose would be damaged that she hadn't even felt labor pains.' Julie once required dental work but 'was terrified the dentist would damage her nose by bumping it while she was anesthetized and that she'd be unaware' that it had been harmed. As a result of that fear, Julie opted to have the procedure without Novocain. Dr Phillips observes that Julie 'preferred the intense physical pain of unanesthetized dental work to the emotional pain of unrecognized nose damage'.

In fact, some patients even use pain as a deterrent, in an attempt to interrupt endless cycles of BDD behaviors. A college student who compulsively trimmed her hair and carried scissors with her constantly to make sure it remained even, told Dr Phillips that she had first tried to throw her scissors away, but when she found herself still unable to resist the urge to cut her hair, she hit her hands with a hammer and intentionally slammed them in a car door.

Opting for physical pain over psychic agony is reminiscent of the intentional patterns of self-injury inflicted by those who cut and burn themselves, even by those who swallow foreign bodies. And yet within BDD, self-harm seems to be a frantic attempt to escape the disease's confines. In chronic self-injury, the act of harm may provide its own form of respite, no matter how fleeting. In BDD the pain brings no such relief. It is the by-product of a despondent effort at making intolerable symptoms abate. And because the actions taken so rarely have any effect on the patient's symptoms, the pain is often suffered in vain.

In this very way, Eddie's endless dermatologic procedures were in vain. BDD, it must be underscored, is a disease of the mind and not the body. Just as a patient's deviated septum would be ill treated by psychotropic medications, so Eddie's trail of cosmetic surgeries utterly failed to diminish any part of his crippling distress. I asked him why, then, he continued to schedule procedure after procedure after procedure.

I half expected him to acknowledge that it must look irrational from my perspective. I thought he might admit to the travesty of saving up months of income only to hand it over, time and again, to treat some invisible scars.

'What else am I supposed to do?' he asked me. 'There's nothing else *to* do. But you know, Doc, there's a stronger laser coming down the pike . . .' And he'd be off, hitching his delusional wagon to the promise of new technology. The next novel treatment. The procedure that this time would really be created to address *his* kind of scarring. This one really, once he had enough money to try it, this one really might work.

Though his fantasies about the future were just that, Eddie was able to accurately describe the trajectory of his past skin treatments and their bearing on his illness. Two-thirds of people who suffer from BDD have an onset of symptoms before they turn eighteen. As someone who first became obsessed with his skin at sixteen, Eddie was right in line with the majority of BDD patients. When he thought about the promise he attached to a dermatologic process, it often carried with it the hope of returning to the more carefree days he remembered from his early adolescence.

'When I learn about a new treatment, I get almost giddy,' he explained to me, 'like I might really have a chance at getting my life back. Like this time things might really change. Then I go into this stretch of frustration and anticipation,' he continued. 'I'm excited and looking forward to the treatment, but I'm frustrated because I can't just go *do* it, you know? I have to save up like crazy before it can happen, and that takes time.' Eddie had gone through so much money chasing perfect skin that he worked extra hours whenever he could in order to keep up with his treatments. He often canceled his appointments with me because he couldn't give up the work time. He had moved in with his sister and her family to save money on rent.

'Once I've got the money and the appointment is scheduled?' he went on. 'That's the only time in my life I feel anything close to happiness. That's like . . .' He paused. 'That's like my one little bit of peace.'

It seemed to me that what Eddie was really talking about was hope. He had been in some form of psychiatric treatment for years, and although his symptoms improved somewhat when he was on the class of antidepressants known as serotonin reuptake inhibitors (SRIs), they didn't fully subside. As he spoke, I realized that the reason the useless surgeries were so reinforcing had nothing to do with their outcomes.

They were addictive because they promised relief, and living with the promise provided a respite from the torture of feeling as if he would always be hideously ugly.

Of course, the promise didn't ever last. 'Right after the procedures, I still feel pretty excited, but I guess that's when the first worries start to creep back in,' Eddie explained. 'What if this last-ditch new laser didn't do what it was supposed to? What if my skin is exactly the same? Or, Jesus Christ, what if it actually looks worse instead of better? For the first couple of days, I can hold on to what the doctor told me: that there'll be redness, or swelling, or whatever. But still I start to see that nothing's really changed. Then . . .' And here Eddie's voice trailed off. He shrugged.

"Then what?' I pressed him.

'Then . . . God. Then it's . . . it's an absolute pit of despair, you know?'

I nodded.

'The money's gone, the excitement is gone . . .'

'The hope?' I asked.

'Yeah,' he said softly. 'Whatever shred of that there was, that's totally blown out of the water. Those are the days, after the procedures don't work like they're supposed to, that I find myself thinking, "You know what? I just need to die."'

Eddie laid out this course as a true expert, familiar with every inch of its terrain. His fluid navigation of it was heartbreaking. That he would subject himself to it over and over again, despite an ability to map it out with utter precision, spoke to . . . what? Some way in which he had been failed by psychiatric treatment? A resistance to healing buried deep within his own mind? My inability to steer him toward safety, toward sanity? The brutality of this disease that would not release its bitter hold?

In writing about what might cause BDD, Dr Phillips gives an explanation that is as maddeningly inexact as my own questions about why

Eddie is trapped in its horrible lockstep. Her explanation feels like grasping. It also is almost certainly true. 'You probably first need to inherit a genetic predisposition to BDD,' she writes. 'This may consist of a vulnerability or susceptibility to developing the disorder BDD specifically or a more general genetic predisposition to worry and obsess – or both. This tendency may involve the brain chemical serotonin and other neurotransmitters, as well as certain areas of the brain. Let's say you're also born with a tendency to have a shy and self-conscious personality; if this temperament is combined with a tendency to obsess and worry, it may further increase your chance of getting BDD. Environmental factors may further increase this biologically based risk; for example, if you're teased a lot as a child or experience lots of rejection, this may further funnel your genetically based worrying tendency and self-consciousness toward BDD symptoms. And if you're already predisposed in these ways to develop BDD, you may be hyperalert to media images of perfection (such as flawless skin) and buy into them more than the average person does. Then, if your boyfriend breaks up with you, that may trigger feelings of inferiority and full-fledged BDD.'

While the consequences of BDD can be grave for patients, the consequences can also be grave for those who treat them. When patients like Eddie have put all their hope and all their money into surgical procedures that do little or nothing to alleviate their symptoms, they conclude that the procedures have failed. Some, like Eddie, internalize that disappointment. Others may hold their physicians accountable for these perceived failures. Sometimes the blaming takes the form of litigiousness. Occasionally it turns violent. A 1996 paper in the medical journal *Dermatologic Clinics* cautions physicians that BDD patients' anger 'may be directed at the attending physician with vitriolic letters, death threats, and even physical violence. In recent times in the United Kingdom', the paper continues, 'one dermatologist and two plastic surgeons have been murdered, and practitioners working in this field should know that there is a small but definite risk of assault when managing these patients. The long and arduous consultations, repeated telephone calls, and constant need for reassurance can put a significant strain on the medical practitioners involved'.

Selma, my patient who sought a dentist to pull all her teeth and 'start over', had not been violent, but she had been threatening. Selma attributed her perceived problems with the appearance of her teeth to the first dental procedure she'd ever had. 'That woman destroyed the alignment of my whole jaw, my bite, everything,' she told me, referring to the technician who had applied a whitening solution to Selma's teeth. That had been more than a decade ago. First, in the months following the procedure, Selma began going to the office to try to confront the technician. She sent letters to the office and to the dentist, threatening lawsuits and blaming the technician for 'ruining' her appearance. Eventually she moved to another part of the country but returned three years later. She immediately went back to the dentist's office, 'to tell that woman what she had put me through since I had seen her last'. When she found that the technician no longer worked there, Selma found her home address and began stalking her, leaving her threatening letters and phone messages. Finally the technician informed the police and got a restraining order against Selma. She complied with the restraining order, but in each of our sessions ten years later she spent at least part of the time ranting about how angry she remained at the woman she blamed for all her unhappiness.

Eddie demonstrated that same persistent adherence to his delusional belief. During the year that I treated him, the frequency of our visits varied dramatically. We were initially scheduled to meet every month, to check in on Eddie's symptoms, to see how the SRI that I had prescribed for him was working. When Eddie admitted he wasn't taking the medicine reliably ('What's the use?' he would say. 'Prozac's not gonna help my acne.') and he found himself thinking more often that he would be better off dead, I saw him on a weekly basis. No matter how frequently or infrequently our appointments were scheduled, Eddie canceled half of them.

When we did meet, I tried every way I could think of to convince him of the potential benefits of cognitive behavioral therapy (CBT), a kind of psychotherapy proven to reduce BDD symptoms, sometimes dramatically. I showed him data about the treatment's efficacy. I told him stories of patients very much like him whom I had treated with SRIs and CBT, and I told him that those patients had escaped the mirror's hold, that they had entered into happier, fuller lives, without surgeries, without suffering.

Eddie remained absolutely certain that I had it all wrong. He believed I saw the same flaws on his body that he did but that I was pretending not to notice and trying to convince him otherwise. His delusion was so deeply entrenched that he *knew* the hideousness of his appearance to be true, as surely as he knew his own name, or his occupation, or his current state of despair.

'I'm not saying that it's not great that those people got better, Dr Montross, it is,' Eddie would say to me. 'It's just that they don't have the skin I have. They don't look like I do.' I tried to talk with Eddie about his reluctance to participate fully in treatment. I tried to cajole him into giving CBT a try. He could see no use in it. 'The problem isn't my thinking, it's my *skin*,' Eddie would say to me over and over. 'Why would I spend time and money on that therapy when I could be working during those extra hours and saving up for the new procedures that will target my real problem?'

Eddie believed so strongly that his problem was dermatologic, not psychiatric, that he saw my treatment – indeed any psychiatric treatment – as misguided at best and deceptive at worst.

He eventually capitulated after I challenged him yet again about his resistance to treatment. 'Maybe your medicines and therapy *could* make me feel better about the way I look,' he allowed. 'But I'd still look the way I do, so I'd be in some medicated state of denial, walking around. Even if I didn't realize it because of the meds or whatever, I'd still be disgusting people with my ugly face.' Eddie was so convinced about his appearance that he feared that medicine or therapy would somehow make him blind to the horrors the rest of the world would see.

When I finished my outpatient year, another psychiatric resident took over the care of all my patients. I recently ran into that psychiatrist, and I asked about Eddie. It seemed that hardly anything about his condition had changed, that he remained plagued by his bodily concerns.

'He's really struggling,' the doctor said. 'There's some new procedure . . . subcision? They put a needle under acne scars to try to break up the connective tissue making the scar, or something. Anyway, he's gotten it done a bunch, even though he's never had any acne scars that I can see.'

I remembered how hard it was to sit with Eddie and manage not to either argue with him about his symptoms or reassure him about them. Dr Phillips repeatedly advised me how little there was to be gained by those actions, so I had always tried to meet him at the level of his sadness, his life losses, his suffering. But it wasn't easy.

'Is he any happier?' I asked his new doctor hopefully.

'I wouldn't say I've ever seen him happy,' the doctor replied. 'I'd say he's absolutely miserable.'

I t is a windless morning in late April, and the sun is shining brightly on Rhode Island's Narragansett Bay. Our friend Welly is staying with us. Deborah has written a play that is up at our regional theater, and Welly has sweetly made the trip from California to see it the night before. I've recently taken up running – about a year in, after two decades of saying I ran only if chased – and Welly and I had planned to go for a jog along the town beach and through the quiet of the neigh-borhood after I dropped the kids off at school. But sometimes the ocean changes things. En route home from the school, there is a rise in the road that dead-ends in a panoramic view of the bay. Lighthouse on the right, bridges to the left, little clam boats anchored in the shallows between on a calm day like this one. The water glimmers sharply in the April light. When I get home, I propose to Welly that we forgo the run and paddle instead. Deborah and I house a borrowed plastic kayak in our garage, and my family members all pitched in at Christmas to give me a stand-up paddleboard, which I have used only once in the cold spring since. When I ask if she'd want to kayak beside me as I paddle, Welly does not hesitate: *Yes.*

The water is frigid, and my body braces as I clamber onto my board, remembering my first outing, during which I fell three times and plunged up to my neck in the freezing bay. But soon I am steady and sure. My legs relax. My arms dip the paddle beneath the surface and, with a satisfying pull, propel me forward. Without discussing it we instinctively head toward the lighthouse. Welly is a sculptor, and as we glide, we chat about her work. She is, it turns out, thinking about the body. How we inhabit the architecture of the bodies we are given. How our bodies can be powerful and how they can be encumbrances. How they can feel inextricably linked to our identities yet how they can also misrepresent and betray us. I am making up some of this in retro-spect, as I too often do about the jobs of my friends, falling captive to their ideas and suddenly following those ideas into thoughts that are more mine than theirs. Still, I think this is the gist of what we said to each other: The body is so innately known and yet still such a mystery. We talk about fidelity, and sex, and superpowers, and Underoos. We cover some territory.

As we're paddling, I bring up BDD: how the mind can believe that the body betrays, when in fact it's the mind that is the guilty party. We head deeper into the bay. It seems fitting that the water grows murkier beneath us. I tell her that I've been doing some thinking about another condition, too. This one has been called apotemnophilia – a not-altogether-accurate term for a condition in which otherwise-sane people want their healthy limbs cut off. From the Greek: *apo-*, 'away from'; *temno-*, 'to cut, hew, maim, wound, or sacrifice'; *-philia*, 'amity, affection, friendship, fondness, liking'. *Having a fondness for cutting away.*

I first became aware of people seeking elective amputations not in my clinical practice but when my friend Jay Baruch, an ER doc and fiction writer, sent me an article that the philosopher and bioethicist Carl Elliott had written on the subject in the *Atlantic*. 'You will want to read this', Jay wrote in the attached message. He knows me.

I say that the term 'apotemnophilia' is not entirely accurate because the suffix '-philia' places these people within a diagnostic classification – the paraphilias – that by definition involves sexual attraction. The *OED* defines a paraphilia as a 'sexual desire regarded as perverted or irregular, specifically attraction to unusual or abnormal sexual objects or practices'. As it turns out, few patients who seek amputations do so for sexual reasons, and even those who acknowledge a sexual component to their desire to become amputees tend to cite another, nonsexual reason as the primary motivating factor. Therefore a new nomenclature has emerged for this condition. A less lovely term, but probably more diagnostically accurate and certainly less potentially pejorative: body integrity identity disorder (BIID).

A person with BIID knows that his limbs are healthy, but he is plagued by the persistent feeling that he is *meant* to be an amputee. He is also not psychotic or hearing voices telling him to cut off his limbs, like the young man winter camping who severed his hand with his hatchet.

In a BBC documentary on the subject entitled *Complete Obsession,* the people seeking amputation do not simply want surgery to remove a body part. They each have a highly specific sense as to where the cut should occur. They describe a sense of their bodies extending beyond where they feel they should. 'It seems that my body stops midthigh on my right leg,' Gregg Furth, a strikingly ordinary-seeming New York psychoanalyst explains. 'The desire that I have,' he says matter-of-factly, "is for an amputation above the knee on the right leg.'

A woman named Corinne in the film repeatedly draws a line with her hands at the crease between her pelvis and her thighs as she tries to explain where she feels her body naturally ends. 'I feel that my legs don't belong to me and they shouldn't be there,' she says, expressing a longing to have them both cut off, 'fairly high' up the thigh.

BIID is not yet included in the *Diagnostic and Statistical Manual of Mental Disorders (DSM)*, though it was suggested for review and consideration for the most recent revision, *DSM*-5. The syndrome is not well understood and is probably quite rare. Yet, as a group, people with these urges are beginning to be studied, and occasionally descriptions appear of patients who may well have suffered from these symptoms in the past. In his meticulously researched book *From Paralysis to Fatigue: A History of Psychosomatic Illness in the Modern Era,* Edward Shorter recounts an incident in 1818 in which 'Benjamin Brodie was invited to consult a "lady in the country on account of a disease of the knee." There were no obvious local findings,' Shorter writes. Brodie 'recommended a course of treatment that failed, and the symptoms became aggravated. "She suffered more than ever, so that she became anxious to undergo the amputation of the limb." Brodie advised against it. "However, her wishes remained unaltered; and two surgeons of eminence in the country, yielding to her entreaties, performed the operation." On completion of the amputation they were surprised to see that they had removed a normal joint.'

Unlike Eddie, and other patients who suffer from body dysmorphic disorder, people with BIID do not want to be rid of their limbs because they perceive them to be hideous, diseased, or faulty in any way. Rather, the limbs feel alien, as if they don't belong. With intact bodies the patients, paradoxically, do not feel whole.

The way in which personal identity seems inextricably linked to the desire for amputation has led to comparisons between BIID and gender dysphoria. In gender dysphoria (previously classified psychiatrically as gender identity disorder and in lay terminology as transsexualism), people experience their gender as different from the one that their physical sex characteristics typically indicate. These syndromes share a disconnect between the fundamental way in which a person feels his identity ought to be and the way that his body *is*. Similarly, people in both groups are subjected to an intense degree of discomfort in their bodies, which may drive them to consider extreme measures to rectify this incongruity.

Gregg Furth and Corinne, like others with BIID, sought out surgeons willing to amputate their healthy legs. Dr Robert Smith, in Scotland, had performed two such procedures in 2000, after which his hospital intervened and forbade him to do any others. In a news conference, Smith told reporters that the elective amputation was 'the most satisfying operation I have ever performed'. Having met with the patients and having determined they were both sane and tormented, he insisted, 'I have no doubt that what I was doing was the correct thing for those patients.' No hospital now permits the elective amputation of healthy limbs.

As a result, people with BIID have turned to their own desperate attempts to become amputees. In 1999 a seventy-nine-year-old man named Philip Bondy paid ten thousand dollars to John Ronald Brown, a surgeon who went to Mexico after he'd had his medical license revoked in the United States for performing black-market sex-change operations in hotel rooms and garages. In return for the money, the surgeon cut off Bondy's healthy leg. Following the surgery Bondy was sent to his hotel room, where he died of gangrene.

Others determined to have limbs amputated have resorted to

gruesome tactics. Arms and legs have been sawn off by chain saws and severed by log splitters or homemade guillotines. People have stretched limbs over tracks in front of oncoming trains. They have packed arms or legs in dry ice for hours and then gone to the hospital, forcing doctors to amputate their irreparably frozen limbs. They have shot hands off with shotguns; they have reached into wood chippers. They deliberately infect wounds; they attempt to burn their limbs beyond repair. A case report in the *Journal of Hand Surgery* described a fifty-one-year-old government employee who first cut his hand off with an axe and then 'proceeded to mutilate the severed part with the axe in order to prevent any possibility of replantation'. As a means both of providing context for such an injury and of educating doctors as to when they might suspect such a condition in one of their patients, the article continues, 'This persistent discomfort and obsession to have a limb amputated can become almost unbearable, and a history of repeated, unexplained injuries to the same segment of the body is common among these patients.'

'I feel my legs don't belong to me and they shouldn't be there,' Corinne says in *Complete Obsession*. 'There is just an overwhelming sense of despair sometimes. I don't want to die, but there are times I don't want to keep living in a body that doesn't feel like mine.'

As with Julie, who endured unanesthetized dental work rather than risk damage to her nose, some people with BIID would rather endure tremendously painful amputation – and the subsequent difficulty of life as an amputee – than continue to live tormented by parts attached to their bodies that feel as if they don't belong.

After I have explained this to Welly as we paddle, this sense of one's own body as alien, the urge of *apo-temno-*, 'to maim, to cut away', I say, 'And here is the unbelievable part . . .'

Welly laughs. '*Here* is the unbelievable part?' she asks. 'Like what came before this is all run-of-the-mill?'

I start giggling, too, but then I lose my balance, so I try to force the look on my face from a silly grin into a stern expression in an attempt to stop laughing. I am terrible at stern expressions. My utter failure at this makes us laugh even harder, and I am so unsteady that I have to kneel on the board to keep from plunging headlong into the deep waters. When we compose ourselves, I paddle beside Welly like that for a while, kneeling. It's quieter somehow. We are on the same level.

'Okay,' I say. 'Let me rephrase. Here is where it gets even more *un*believable.' She nods, listening. 'Surgery makes them better.'

'Wait . . . what?' Welly stammers. 'What do you *mean*?'

'Yeah,' I say. 'The people who amputate their limbs feel better. It's not like body dysmorphic disorder, where a delusional preoccupation continues. For years and years, these people feel like they have an extra limb that doesn't belong to them. They feel like they're meant to be amputees. And once they finally are, they feel relief. Resolution. Cured.'

Welly gapes, then starts to nod, and eventually we keep talking. We return to possible parallels between elective amputation and gender-reassignment surgery, how maybe surgery in both instances is the exterior righting of some kind of long-endured internal wrong.

I stand back up on the paddleboard. I stand on my own strong legs, and I feel my arms at work as they pull the paddle through the water. The spring sun glints off of my skin, and I do not worry how I look. I feel the rays and how they warm me. My body – all of it: my limbs, my mind, my sex – it is who I am. Its imperfections are mine, too, and they do not consume me. By what alignment of neurochemistry and circumstance have I been granted that solid balance?

Medical research is beginning to explore how best to treat patients with BIID. Though they acknowledge that the evidence available is 'scant', Tim Bayne and Neil Levy confirm in a paper in the

Journal of Applied Philosophy that those 'who succeed in procuring an amputation seem to experience a significant and lasting increase in well-being" and "do not develop the desire for additional amputations'.

In *Whole,* a 2003 documentary about patients with BIID, the people who have undergone amputation express precisely these kinds of sentiments. A man who packed his leg in dry ice, inducing severe frostbite that necessitated amputation, explained, 'The feeling overall is of rebirth. Instantaneously, from that point, when I woke from the anesthetic, all my torment had disappeared.' Another man, who shot his leg off with a shotgun, saw no alternative course of action. 'What I did,' he explains, 'was absolutely imperative. The alternative that day was suicide. . . . My only regret was that it didn't happen sooner.' A third man, one of Dr Robert Smith's elective-surgical amputees, describes himself postsurgery as 'normal now . . . relaxed, comfortable, at ease. [I] only get stressed out by things at work and other pressures like everybody else. I don't have this additional big burden sitting on my shoulders. . . . By taking a leg away, I've actually been made more complete. I'm actually more of a person than I was before.'

A recently published paper by Rianne Blom and her colleagues at the University of Amsterdam found similar results from a questionnaire she administered to 54 individuals with BIID. 'Actual amputation of the limb was effective in all 7 cases who had surgical treatment', she writes. 'Amputation of the healthy body part appears to result in remission of BIID and an impressive improvement of quality of life.' One responder inadvertently revealed as much when he or she wrote, 'I'm wondering if I am eligible to participate in this study, because since my amputation I do not have BIID feelings anymore.'

How, then, as doctors, do we proceed? A surgical procedure exists that appears to alleviate the anguish of people who are truly suffering. In attempts to treat the condition, medications have proved ineffective, and psychotherapy, as the British psychiatrist Russell Reid has put it, 'doesn't make a scrap of difference in these people'. At present no treatment exists that we know of that is anywhere near as helpful as the surgery.

And yet. As doctors we have – all of us – sworn an oath to first do no harm. There is no more visceral sense of what constitutes harm than cutting off a healthy hand or severing two healthy legs from the torso they support. It is, Bayne and Levy assert, this visceral reaction – more than objective medical decision making – that has resulted in the unwillingness of any hospital to permit elective amputation.

Bayne and Levy acknowledge a 'sense of repugnance that is evoked by the idea that a person might wish to rid themselves of an apparently healthy limb'. But they caution us against mistaking our repugnance for clinical – or even ethical – judgment: 'Disgust responses can alert us to the possibility that the practices in question *might* be morally problematic, but they do not seem to be reliable indicators of moral transgression.'

Nonetheless, our repugnance leads us to call into question the autonomy of those who request such a procedure. And hence we refuse to do the thing they ask of us. We argue that they are requesting unethical and unnecessary medical treatment. We say that they are choosing elective disability over present health. We decide they do not have a right to the procedures they seek.

There are undeniable costs of disability that reach beyond the responsibility of the amputee. People without limbs require different levels of assistance to navigate the world, from simple crutches to sophisticated wheelchairs. Homes and cars must be modified. For reasons that are not completely understood, lower-limb amputees are at increased risk of cardiovascular disease. As a society we have determined that insurance companies and government programs should pay for medical care and supplies for conditions – such as emphysema from smoking cigarettes or joint replacements caused by obesity – that are arguably just as self-determined. But in the case of elective amputation, to whom should the costs of care fall?

The medical ethicist Art Caplan has argued that the disturbing nature of the request is in and of itself adequate evidence that people who wish to be amputees should not be granted autonomy to amputate their limbs. 'It's absolute, utter lunacy to go along with a request to maim somebody', he has said. 'The cure is not to yield to the illness and conform to the obsession. And this is not just about "do no harm". It's also about whether [patients] are competent to make a decision when they're running around saying, "Chop my leg off."'

However, no matter how upsetting the potential outcome, the legal concept of autonomy requires only that a person have an adequate understanding of the likely consequences of an action. A Jehovah's Witness may refuse a blood transfusion if she can demonstrate that she fully understands she may die without one. And we permit patients to undertake any number of surgical procedures that carry with them real risks, real consequences, and not one iota of medical necessity or even benefit. In his piece in the *Atlantic,* Carl Elliott gets at this logical breach. He admits being swayed by the 'simple, relentless logic to [the] requests for amputation. . . . "I am suffering," they tell me', he writes. '"I have nowhere else to turn." They realize that life as an amputee will not be easy. They understand the problems they will have with mobility, with work, with their social lives. . . . [But] they are willing to pay their own way. Their bodies belong to them, they tell me. The choice should be theirs. What is worse: to live without a leg or to live with an obsession that controls your life? For at least some of them, the choice is clear – which is why they are talking about chain saws and shotguns and railroad tracks. And to be honest, haven't surgeons made the human body fair game? You can pay a surgeon to suck fat from your thighs, lengthen your penis, enlarge your breasts, redesign your labia, even . . . implant silicone horns in your forehead or split your tongue like a lizard's. Why not amputate a limb?'

I am inclined to agree, but I can't deny that I feel great discomfort in doing so. I, too, feel repugnance at the idea of someone's choosing to cut off a limb. I fear that elective amputation may be a misguided treatment – treating a symptom without understanding the disease from which it comes. This is not a break across bone that causes the leg to give, not an atherosclerotic plaque that dislodges from its vessel wall to block the blood flow to the brain. This is not known cause and seen effect. It is mysterious origins and symptoms that are difficult to try to comprehend.

And yet so much of medicine – and hence so much of psychiatry – dwells in exactly this space. We do not understand why schizophrenic patients are plagued by visions and voices. We do not know why some deep depressions do not relent. We do not know which precise factors take root to give rise to the compulsions of BDD. But we offer treatment – which, to varying degrees, is not entirely benign – nonetheless. We try to alleviate suffering even if we don't fully understand the mechanisms of what we prescribe. We do what we can. As the author of one journal article succinctly wrote of elective amputation for BIID, 'No alternative means of relieving suffering exists.'

In order to determine whether there are any other treatments for BIID, we must have a better sense of the origin of the disorder. There have been countless theories put forth to attempt to explain how BIID could arise. They range from the psychodynamic (perhaps the patient lacked parental love as a child and longs to be an amputee because he subconsciously views amputees as people who are given attention and sympathy, which his childhood lacked) to the biologic (in the same way that sea cucumbers, reptiles, and spiders may sacrifice a limb when threatened, so, too, might human beings). For the most part, the theories strike me as very creative and not very plausible.

However, we may be on the cusp of beginning to understand more. There are similarities between BIID and some specific neurological conditions. Patients with somatoparaphrenia, whose name implies a dysjunction between body (*somato-*) and mind (*-phrenia*), have specific delusions. They believe that their own body parts are in fact parts of the bodies of others. These patients often confabulate, or invent stories, to shore up their assertions. A case report recently published in the *Journal of Neurological Sciences,* for example, described a woman who believed that her own hand was in fact that of her sister. She made up poems about seeking her own lost hand and even joked that her sister should pay for parking for her hand, since it was in the patient's bed.

Asomatognosia (*a-*, meaning 'no or without'; *somato-*, 'body or bodily'; *-gnosia,* 'knowledge') is a lack of awareness of ownership of one's limb. An asomatognostic patient may perceive his own leg to belong to the doctor, for instance, but unlike with somatoparaphrenic patients, once the asomatognostic's error is pointed out to him, he is able to understand – even if only temporarily – that the limb is in fact his own.

In contrast to patients with somatoparaphrenia and asomatognosia, people with BIID are not delusional and they do recognize their limbs as their own, though they do not feel that it should be so. Nonetheless, this triad of conditions may well be linked through neuroanatomy. Somatoparaphrenia and asomatognosia often result from strokes that leave areas of the brain damaged. Many studies implicate dysfunction of a particular part of the brain – the parietal lobe – in these syndromes, and there is now some evidence that BIID may also arise from this neurological territory.

A 2011 paper by Anna Sedda in *Neuropsychology Review* cites an experiment conducted by Paul D. McGeoch at the University of California, San Diego. McGeoch and his colleagues tapped on the feet of a group of patients with BIID and those of a control group of healthy patients. Using magnetoencephalography – a means of measuring electrical currents in the brain – McGeoch et al. found that tapping healthy people's feet on either side evoked electrical activity in the parietal lobe of the brain. However, when they tapped the feet of BIID patients on the side where they desired an amputation, that same electrical response was absent. McGeoch and his colleagues concluded that

'BIID is caused by a failure to represent, partially or fully, one or more limbs in the right-superior parietal lobe.' In other words, the brain doesn't sense that the 'foreign' limbs are there in the same way it senses the limbs that feel more normally integrated into the person's body, and identity. Or, as Corinne said, 'I feel that my legs don't belong to me and they shouldn't be there.'

If BIID were truly demonstrated to have neurological origins, it might be perceived as more legitimate. Maybe then the symptoms would still strike us all as unbelievable, but the people who suffer from the disorder would no longer be seen that way. Like somatoparaphrenia or asomatognosia, whose associated stroke lesions can be confirmed by brain imaging, the desire to amputate a limb might then become yet another of the baffling ways in which our minds can misfire. Perhaps, as a culture that more easily legitimizes illnesses for which we believe there is a structural or chemical cause, we would then be more forgiving of the people trapped in this web of the brain's discrepancies.

Still, what do we *do* for the woman who wants her legs off? For the man who wishes to amputate his hand? Does the fact that there may be a neurological origin for their symptoms make it more compelling to honor their requests because we now understand whence they come? Or does it make it more misguided – even abhorrent – to do so? Why would we operate on someone's healthy leg to treat a disorder of the parietal lobe of her brain?

How do we, as doctors, define 'help'? How do we define 'harm'?

Two months after Deborah and I move with our three- and five-year-old children to a home near the ocean, a hurricane strikes. We have followed our experienced neighbors' direction in the days before the storm: In came bird feeders and deck chairs, in came wind chimes, in came anything that could be sent blasting through a window. The houses on the water have large sheets of plywood nailed over their windows and doors. We buy water and candles and nonperishables. We check our flashlights. We hunker down. We wait.

The winds begin late Friday. Early Saturday morning, as I drive to the hospital to work, the sky is a dark gray-green and trees are already whipping angrily about. The radio has warned that it is an 'astronomical high tide'. I don't know what that means technically, but I see that it means water from the estuary is already lapping over the road. When I drive through the water, a thick fan of droplets launches out from either side of my car.

Nurses and patients and I all watch out the windows that morning as the heavy winds and rains come. I call Deborah every half hour. The winds are intense, she says. She and the kids are watching movies holed up in the basement. When do I think I could come home?

I round quickly and type notes that are briefer than usual. In the middle of writing my orders, the hospital goes black. A few seconds later, the emergency generator kicks in and the lights are back on, but a maintenance worker brings a cart full of flashlights up to the unit just in case. My pager goes off; I glance at the numbers on the screen and see it is the numeric code Deborah and I have that means 'Call home'. I do. It rings and rings. I try her cell phone. She answers.

'The power is out,' she says. 'And the wind is really howling.' She hesitates, then says softly, 'Babe, come home.'

The winds reach more than eighty miles per hour in our neighborhood. Tree limbs lash against one another, then tear from their trunks and are flung by the wind across roads, across yards, across power lines. As I drive home, streets are blocked by massive fallen trees, their splintered stumps raised up into the sky as if in protest. Cables dangle from telephone poles onto sidewalks. As I cross a bridge over an inlet, the few boats that have not been taken in to safety before the storm are being tossed roughly by the ocean like little bobbing bath toys.

When I finally walk in the door of our house, Deborah exhales. She looks pale but has a forced smile on her face that I recognize from turbulence on planes – she is terrified, but she doesn't want the children to be. And it has worked. They run up to me shrieking about what fun it is to be 'camping' in the basement, and how cool the sounds of the wind are, and that Mommy has given them each their own flashlight to use, isn't that amazing?

It is, I say, and pull Deborah close to me. The rest of the day, despite the unrelenting gusts, the cracking of limbs, the hammer of rain, she is not scared. She swears there was something exceptional about the wind's strength while I was gone. That may be. Or else there may be a way in which it is scarier to face a threat alone, without someone there to see what you are experiencing, to comfort, to understand.

When the winds finally relent a bit and the radio says the worst has passed, we step outside. The ground is entirely green with leaf litter, and branches are down as far as the eye can see. Our house is unscathed, but our neighbors, Jim and Wendy, aren't so lucky. A huge tree from their front yard has been uprooted and has landed on their roof. Another has fallen across their driveway and is resting on their car. That evening we go for a walk with the kids to look around. Jim is standing beside the tree.

'We can't believe this, Jim. We're so sorry!' Deborah says. 'What a nightmare for you.'

'Oh, this?' Jim smiles. 'Hey, come on in, you guys.' He gestures for us to follow him, and as we duck beneath the branches hanging over his front door, we see that their home is packed full of our neighbors. In an instant, someone hands me a cup of wine and someone else gives our kids plates of mac and cheese. A generator hums in the backyard, and the kitchen counter is covered in food. We look at Wendy with confusion.

'I'm from New Orleans.' She beams. 'When this kind of thing happens, you throw a party. That's how you move forward.' Deborah and I look at each other in shock. 'Do y'all want some chili?' Wendy asks.

In the hours after the hurricane, Narragansett Bay is transformed. Mighty, loping swells crash in the shallows, scraping the beach and carving great craters in the sand. Along the beach far into the distance, star fish of every size have been thrown up by the waves. They are all dead, or dying. I don't know why. Were I seeing this body of water for the first time, I would be unable to imagine it as placid as it was the day that Welly and I paddled alongside each other.

The circumstances of the world shift without explanation or warning. Why do some of us meet difficulty with despair and others do so with fortitude? Who can comfort us when we are scared? Whom do we gather around us when darkness descends and the trees fall? What if a tragedy in a person's life cannot be so plainly seen by others? What if it cannot be understood at all?

CHAPTER THREE

Your Drugs Take Away the Love

I remember when I lost my mind
There was something so pleasant about that place
Even your emotions have an echo in so much space
And when you're out there without care
Yeah, I was out of touch
But it wasn't because I didn't know enough
I just knew too much.
Does that make me crazy?
Possibly.

– Gnarls Barkley, 'Crazy'

Late nights in the psychiatric emergency room, it's not unusual to meet someone who claims to be Jesus. The night that I first saw Colin, the patients had been relatively ordinary by psych-ER standards: a demented elderly man who kept asking me to lie down in his reclining chair with him, a fifty-something-year-old woman withdrawing from alcohol, a forty-five-year-old lawyer and father of two who had been so depressed that he wanted to drive his car off a bridge. I was working on the inpatient wards at the time, but I had picked up the night shift in the ER because the hospital needed extra staffing.

I was typing my assessment of the suicidal lawyer when Colin wandered through the metal detector, past the blood-pressure cuff and Breathalyzer, and up to the doorway of the ER's administrative area, where he stood staring straight at me. At first I felt the sensation of eyes on me. Then, when I turned to find the source of the feeling, I saw Colin: a young man, maybe in his early twenties. His skin was tanned. He had long, tousled, light brown hair that had been sun-bleached to blond in streaks, and he was wearing an embroidered white tunic smudged with dirt. Unlike the many patients I encountered who claimed to be Jesus, this guy actually looked the part.

When my own glance met his stare, there was no self-conscious shift of his gaze, no quick turn away. Instead his eyes continued to bore straight into mine. His face was expressionless and haunting. Eventually one of the security guards gently guided him back into the waiting area. I finished typing and began to interview another patient. The next time I walked through the waiting area, Colin was gone.

Frequently when I leave a shift in the ER, cases and clinical questions from the night linger in my mind. *Did I double-check the lab work on the demented patient to rule out a delirium-inducing infection? Was the woman who had been cutting the insides of her thighs with a razor blade really safe enough to go home?* This night the image of Colin's fixed stare stayed with me as I left the hospital.

In general, psychiatrists don't scare easy. We become accustomed to patients telling us that their thoughts will kill us as they've killed nations, that they know we are part of a conspiracy to place satellites in their houses and that we will have to be brought to justice. Sometimes I've been uncomfortable enough to bring a security guard into the room with me – as when an enormous man who had spent a decade incarcerated for murder was released from prison, caught a bus straight to the psychiatric hospital, and told me that the red eye that had commanded him to kill was hovering around the room in which he and I were talking. But more typically these stories are the ones we share with our colleagues whose shifts begin as ours end and who ask how the night was. Nonetheless, something about Colin's silent intensity had unnerved me, and, not knowing whether he'd been admitted or released, I found myself skittishly looking around, half expecting to see him as I walked to my car to drive home.

The next morning I went into the locked inpatient ward where I worked during the days and gathered my patients' charts. Because patient stays are short in the era of managed, and largely outpatient, mental-health care, on any given day my stack of charts included a fair number of patients whose names were new to me. Other charts belonged to terribly familiar faces: patients whose telling 'episode number', designating how many times they had previously been hospitalized, could easily be more than twice their age. (The most recent of these examples that I encountered – a sixty-five-year-old man caught in a chronic cycle of homelessness and suicidality – was on his 246th episode.)

On the unit I'd typically situate myself with the charts in one of the small private interview rooms. While a medical student would go rouse a patient from her bed and usher her into the room to talk, I'd skim quickly over the evaluation done at admission so I would have an idea of the circumstances that had brought the patient to the point of psychiatric hospitalization.

This morning was no different. The med student said, 'I'll start with Room 32B,' and walked out. I picked up the corresponding chart, flipped it open, and saw the three-inch-by-three-inch admission photograph of Colin, eyes staring into the camera as intently as he'd been staring into the administrative work space of the ER, just as intently as he'd been staring at me.

Late nights during residency training – or early mornings after we'd worked twelve, twenty-four, even thirty hours straight – my fellow residents and I would sometimes make a game of those snapshots. They're universally grainy and off center, taken by a camera attached to the hospital's intake computer, but the shared belief of all psychiatric residents is that the further along one gets in one's training, the more likely one is to be able to determine a patient's precise diagnosis by merely looking at the picture. It's a ridiculous assertion, of course, which elucidates the stereotypes we develop as doctors more than it does any consistently discernible physical traits of mental illness. Still, we play the game.

Those admission photos – and the assumptions we make about them – are a perfect example of how certain realms of medicine can come to be devoid of empathy. Countless factors in medical education contribute to allowing a young doctor's empathy to fade. Residents may legally work as many as eighty hours per week; that kind of ongoing sleep deprivation in the midst of such emotionally demanding work can turn even the most humane doctor into an inattentive grouch. As doctors, we must also find ways to protect ourselves from the aspects of our patients' conditions that upset us, so that we are not overcome by the onslaught of suffering in which we practice. Sometimes we do this in healthy ways – we talk with loved ones or therapists, we run or play music or cook, we dwell on the gratitude we have for our own relatively healthy lives. Other times we rely too heavily on alcohol, or we immerse ourselves entirely in work to the exclusion of every other element of our lives, or we burn out, or we quit. Still other times we find immature but relatively harmless means of diversion. Like the narratives we invent about our patients' photographs.

When I see Colin's snapshot at the front of his chart, I hear in my mind an imagined banter between residents:

'On the run from the Branch Davidians' compound. And angry about the government raid, which he feels interfered with his ascension to join the Hale-Bopp comet or whatever bullshit that was,' one resident would begin.

'Ooooh, that's good,' the other would reply. 'Diagnosis?'

'He's all Axis I. Delusional disorder. Maybe with some intermittent explosive disorder mixed in to account for the uncontrollable anger. You want to agree and give up now, or do you have a better theory?'

'Nope. Listen to this: first psychotic break, exacerbated by heavy pot use and occasional assorted hallucinogens. Mostly 'shrooms. He thinks he's Jesus and is receiving personal messages from God. He believes he can see through to our souls, and he doesn't like what he sees.'

'Okay, diagnosis?'

'Too soon to say. He'll get Axis I: Psychosis NOS. And then in six months, when it's lasted long enough to meet criteria, he'll be schizophrenic, like some uncle on his mom's side who lived in the hospital for thirty years.'

And then, to lay any snap judgments to rest, I read Colin's emergency-room evaluation.

'Patient's Chief Complaint: "There is a good energy here." History of the Present Illness: Patient is a twenty-three-year-old male who was brought to the hospital by his girlfriend secondary to an increase in bizarre behavior. The patient eloped from the emergency department and was brought back by the police. Patient's girlfriend describes odd behavior at home, including walking backward and walking in a circle before picking an item up, both of which the patient explains as actions that "untrack energy". The patient has also urinated in a Coke bottle and says he is "sleeping without sleeping". Patient has refused meds from his psychiatrist, whom he has seen twice weekly for the past six weeks. He says he is having trouble expressing his thoughts and that "I have a lot of things I need to accomplish." Patient's parents arrived from Chicago after they were called by patient's girlfriend. They report that they believe he has "had a spiritual awakening and wants to be a better person", but they agree that his behavior is concerning.' Finally, on the bottom of the page, the doctor who had done the evaluation had scrawled a quote from Colin: 'I am functioning normally. I don't know why people think I'm not.'

The medical student walked in and gestured for Colin – still dressed in his stained tunic – to follow. He did, and stared at me again with the familiar gaze from the night before. Then he stared with the same intensity at the empty chair to my left, then at the locked window with no shade, and finally at the Monet poster encased in plastic and bolted to the wall. When asked to, he sat. And smiled.

'Hi Colin, I'm Dr Montross,' I said, 'and you've already met Vijay, the medical student on our team. If it's okay with you, I'm going to let Vijay start, and then I might pipe in at the end with a few more questions. How does that sound?'

'Sure,' replied Colin. And then to Vijay, he said, 'Welcome.' I could tell that the student wasn't exactly sure how to respond.

'Uh . . . thanks,' Vijay stammered. 'Why don't we start by hearing why it is that you came to the hospital?'

Colin sat quietly for what was probably a minute but seemed like much more. Then, right when I was on the verge of repeating Vijay's question, the silence broke.

'I'm having trouble communicating my life journey to others,' Colin said.

'Tell me what you mean by that,' Vijay asked, leaning forward in his chair.

'Well,' Colin responded, smiling, 'I think you know this.'

Vijay smiled back, perplexed, then shrugged.

Colin continued. 'The most important thing for all of us to know is that life is joy. I'm experiencing a soulful happiness, and I think it is hard for everyone to comprehend.'

As the interview went on, I jotted my own rough clinical assessment for the file: 'Wide-eyed, malodorous young man in tunic, unshaven.

Speech is slow. Thought process is disorganized and circumstantial; content is grandiose. Patient denies auditory or visual hallucinations but does endorse elated mood. Affect is expansive. Insight and judgment are poor, as evidenced by the fact that patient does not see the need for help.'

Vijay finished gathering some final information. Colin had graduated from a prestigious university with an art degree; his senior thesis had been a series of huge metal sculptures. Since college he had been employed on and off as a metalworker on construction sites to support his artwork. He had recently quit to spend a month following a woman called Amma the Hugging Saint through the western mountains of the United States. Amma's doctrine is love, he told me. She feels love for all people, and she provides comfort to those who suffer by hugging and blessing them. During the time he was with Amma, Colin *had* smoked pot and used some hallucinogens, but he said there had been no drug use for a month or more, and his clean toxicology screen from admission supported this claim.

I had a list of potential diagnoses in mind. My first thought had been drugs, but given the results of the toxicology screen, that etiology was rather convincingly out. There was a remote chance that his symptoms were the result of exposure to some volatile substance in his metalwork, but his blood tests weren't indicative of any kind of dangerous solvent or heavy-metal exposure. The other two options were either bipolar mania or a primary psychotic disorder like schizophrenia. In both of those conditions, medication would be the treatment of choice for an acute flare of symptoms like this one.

'Colin, thank you so much for sharing your thoughts with us,' I said. 'I know you've felt misunderstood recently, so we're going to work very hard to understand what you're experiencing.' This was true, but it was also an attempt to navigate the complexities of trying to treat someone exhibiting psychotic symptoms without reaching too far into paternalism or, worse, trickery. Frequently patients are reticent to take medication. Sometimes their reasons are good and sound ones. Sometimes their fears are paranoid, their beliefs are illogical, or their minds simply cannot process the information fully enough to make an informed decision. I believed that medication could help Colin, and as a result I tried to convince him to give it a try. I thought my best strategy was to talk to him about it in his own terms. 'We have some medicines that I think could help you communicate that experience more clearly.'

Colin looked at me quizzically. 'Why would I take medicine?' he asked. 'I'm in love with the feeling I have right now. This joy is better than any drugs.'

And this is how our conversations went that morning and for the next few mornings. The nursing notes in the chart were similar from one shift to the next: 'Patient is pleasant. Dreamy and detached. He continues to pace on the unit or stand in place until redirected. Refusing meds.' A few days in, during our morning session, Colin began asking to leave.

'It's not that there isn't plenty to love in here,' he said, gesturing toward a metal filing cabinet and then an institutional plastic chair. 'But I'm not sure how much longer this place needs me.' And here is where things for Colin – and for me – became a good deal more complicated than they already were.

Colin had been brought into the hospital involuntarily. In every state in America, a physician may commit a patient to psychiatric care against his will if the doctor believes there is an imminent danger that the patient will harm himself or others. The work of Dr Paul Christopher, my colleague at Brown, has called attention to the fact that the consequences of hospitalizing someone against his will vary widely from one state to the next. In Rhode Island, where we practice, once a patient is involuntarily committed, he can be hospitalized against his will for up to ten days before a court hearing is mandated. Many states allow fewer days, but some allow far more. In West Virginia a patient may be held against his will for only one day; in Georgia no hearing is required until twenty days of inpatient hospitalization have passed.

Plus, even in the absence of imminent danger, many states allow a physician to commit a patient against his will if he is classified as 'gravely disabled'. In 1975 the Supreme Court asserted in *O'Connor v. Donaldson* that the inability to care for oneself does not sufficiently demonstrate danger unless survival is at stake. 'A State', the court ruled, 'cannot constitutionally confine . . . a non-dangerous individual who is capable of surviving safely in freedom by himself or with the help of willing and responsible family members or friends.'

Colin's emergency certification form cited this exact sort of 'grave disability': 'Patient not eating, not drinking adequate fluids. Delusional. Periods of bizarre posturing. Twenty-pound weight loss in six to eight weeks.' And with that he was in.

It's not a stretch to say that simply by virtue of his position, Colin was powerless to a certain degree. We had the legal right to keep him inpatient for ten days. As long as he did not take any of the medications we offered, we had little grounds upon which to discharge him. Colin was caught in a circle of logic. If he continued to deny that he had a mental illness that was in need of treatment, we could continue to assert that his insight and judgment were impaired and that therefore we had cause to hold him against his will.

It's easy in a situation such as Colin's to regard the institution of psychiatry as the authoritarian legacy of *One Flew Over the Cuckoo's Nest,* to think of psychiatrists as cartoonish egomaniacs who thrive on their ability to take away the agency of others or who leave no room for divinity, for difference. Indeed, many patients who are admitted to my care reveal deep-seated fears that they will be stripped of their rights, medicated against their will, restrained, or sedated into the 'Thorazine shuffle'.

Yet in reality, psychiatrists, like their colleagues who go into various other medical specialties, have a specific desire to help people heal and to treat them humanely in that pursuit. And so behind all the posturing and joking about our patients' admission photographs is the hope that we really are honing our diagnostic abilities and, in doing so, might be able to lead a patient out of the throes of depression or the haunted hallways of psychosis.

When involuntary hospitalizations come into play, it is almost always because study after study demonstrates that we, as doctors, are terrible at predicting which of our patients – be they depressed or delusional – will kill themselves. And in a profession whose every aim is to heal and help, the assurance of protection often feels more precious than the preservation of autonomy. Without a crystal ball to show us which patients will be safe and which will not, we must rely on our clinical intuition. We meet patients for perhaps thirty minutes and must in that period of time determine whether they are telling us the truth, whether they are able to follow a safety plan, or whether they are impulsive enough – or disturbed enough – to jump off a bridge or push a bystander in front of a train. We have no medical imaging that will tell us the answer, no blood test to shore up our clinical intuition.

It may be tempting to lament the medication of a patient's heightened sense of connectedness or of his new spiritual fervor. Indeed, Colin's case was even more ambiguous because he seemed to be more elated than distressed, yet the costs and dangers associated with psychosis are tragically real. The famed author and neurologist Oliver Sacks points out the perilous allure of madness in discussing what he calls euphoric 'hyperstates' or states of 'ominous extravagance'. Sacks cautions us against ignoring – or, worse, celebrating – symptoms that seem to be happy but are a departure from the person's typical self: 'The paradox of an illness which can present as wellness – as a wonderful feeling of health and well-being, and only later reveal its malignant potentials – is one of the chimeras, tricks and ironies of nature.' In fact, a heightened 'good' feeling – what George Eliot evocatively called 'dangerous wellness' – can itself be a signal of sickness to come, more terrible still for its deception. Most of us cannot exist over time in a sustained state of exultation. More often a high is a sign of a crash to come. Many of the healthiest among us are familiar with that truth. For the mentally ill, the danger can be even more pronounced. The poet Robert Lowell, who endured both the excoriating manias and the debilitating depressions of bipolar illness, wrote, 'If we see a light at the end of the tunnel, / it's the light of an oncoming train.'

The persistent *One Flew Over the Cuckoo's Nest* mythology about psychiatry has doctors forcibly overmedicating and overtreating people who require neither medication nor treatment. The opposite is true. Far more often the most ill patients struggle to obtain access to treatment and to maintain their adherence to medication. Far more often the mentally ill among us are undertreated. And the consequences of untreated mental illness – from financial ruin and homelessness to violence and suicide – can be truly grave.

I had seen countless patients who had endured the consequences and indignities of untreated mania or psychosis. A man who suddenly felt an intense connection to nature left his home to live in the woods off Interstate 95. He drank daily from a pond of stagnant water, inducing diarrheal illness and eventually life-threatening dehydration. A manic businessman in a euphoric frenzy gambled away his company's assets and his family's entire savings before he acquiesced to treatment. A paranoid young man stabbed and mildly injured an elderly stranger for no apparent reason. When the police arrested him at his home, the man's girlfriend cautioned them to be careful, explaining that he had recently been psychotic and dangerous. Once at the station, the man grabbed the gun of the interrogating officer, fired multiple times, killing the officer, and then jumped out a third-story window.

Once apprehended, the man was beaten by the police until he was disfigured and was eventually sentenced to two consecutive life terms in prison.

I felt that if Colin were left untreated, he would be at risk for these kinds of dire consequences, yet he did not share my concern. Eventually he began taking our medicine, but only after I asked him why, if he loved all that was of the world, he would not also love these small blue pills. I'm not sure how much of his agreement had to do with my colluding argument and how much with his growing understanding that going along with the treatment plan would speed up his discharge.

After a day or two of the antipsychotics, the nursing notes reflect a subtle change: 'Patient more lucid; states he is communicating more clearly. Patient also states he no longer feels the love he once did from inanimate objects. The patient is less grandiose, more subdued. Sometimes seems confused.'

Colin did not say that he was sad in the wake of his euphoria, but he certainly did not seem particularly relieved either. He was sleeping regularly, and eating, and consistently urinating in the bathroom, signs that were reassuring to me. Still, the ecstasy that he seemed to have been feeling was less prominent, if it was there at all. One morning as we met, Colin stared at the floor, solemn. 'I'm not sure about this existence,' he said to me. 'Are you?'

I gave him the nebulous diagnosis of Psychosis, Not Otherwise Specified. I knew that Colin could be in a psychotic episode within the context of bipolar illness, but I worried he might be in the early stages of schizophrenia. His age fit both possible diagnoses. Half of all cases of bipolar illness emerge before the age of twenty-five; the average age of onset of schizophrenia for men is the early to mid-twenties. Bipolar disorder is more than twice as prevalent in the United States as schizophrenia, affecting 2.6 percent of the adult population as opposed to 1.1 percent, so by numbers alone it was more likely for a young man like

Colin to be afflicted with bipolar disorder. Still, schizophrenia's fearsome specter loomed in my mind, partially because Colin's symptoms strongly matched the description for the illness's onset and partially because the consequences of such a diagnosis – unlike those of bipolar disorder – had such catastrophic implications.

The *DSM* describes the first indications of schizophrenic illness – the 'prodromal phase' – as a 'slow and gradual development of a variety of signs and symptoms (e.g., social withdrawal, loss of interest in school or work, deterioration in hygiene and grooming, unusual behavior, outbursts of anger)'. I thought of Colin's on-and-off metalwork, the initial ER description of him as 'malodorous . . . unshaven', his girlfriend's concern, his parents' characterization of this period of time as a kind of spiritual awakening. 'Family members may find this behavior difficult to interpret', the *DSM* continues, and may 'assume that the person is "going through a phase."'

If Colin was in the midst of this prodromal phase, then his disorganized behavior – walking backward, urinating in Coke bottles – would continue and his odd beliefs about file cabinets emanating love would bloom into full-fledged delusions. He might begin to hear voices. He might withdraw from his girlfriend and his family. He might become paranoid instead of euphoric. But he would need to have these symptoms for six months in order to meet criteria for schizophrenia. Only time would clarify whether my fears were true.

A round the time I treated Colin, I traveled to an interdisciplinary conference on the theme of madness in order to present a paper. My fellow presenters were an eclectic and interesting group. I was one of only three psychiatrists. There were a handful of psychologists and social workers, but the majority of speakers and attendees were academics in the humanities who studied madness in literature, or in linguistics, or from a sociological perspective, or within history. There were also a small number of patients at the conference who self-identified as 'survivors' of mental illness or as 'mental-health consumers', a term meant to empower patients by placing them in a reciprocal position with mental-health providers. Within their ranks were representatives of Mad Pride and people from the antipsychiatry movement.

In general, I like a good discussion, and there were plenty over the course of this three-day conference. As at any such event, several of the presentations were fascinating and several were dull. Yet as the conference progressed, I found myself first becoming dubious about some of the papers presented, and then finally I began to get downright furious.

It seemed that particularly among university academicians, the urge to render madness romantic was strong. *Isn't it so,* they argued, *that passion is a kind of madness? That it is from a crazed and not-commonly-understood state that the most vivid and intensely human art emerges?* One after another they began to list, in an attempt to bolster this argument, a chorus of names that have come to symbolize both great torment and great genius: *Woolf,* they said, *Dante, Sexton, Lowell.* With each pronouncement the group seemed to gain confidence and momentum: *Shelley, Plath, van Gogh.* It struck me as a marching song. A cadence by which the Mad Pride parade could rally and process: *Handel, Hemingway, Munch!*

I was uneasy and annoyed with the emphasis on the creative benefits of madness, though admittedly, at times, those who are stricken by their visions or mercurial moods seem to be the strongest proponents of this perspective. And who knows better than they? 'As an experience', Virginia Woolf once declared, 'madness is terrific I can assure you, and not to be sniffed at; and in its lava I still find most of the things I write about.' To top it off, the allure of Woolf's 'madness' is not limited to this heady state of inspiration but also offers a kind of rare and perfect productivity. 'It shoots out of one everything shaped, final', she professed, 'not in mere driblets, as sanity does'.

It is both difficult to argue against the authority of such a statement and difficult to *want* to argue against the truth of it. There is something magical about an idea like this, and something explanatory. We, in our hemmed-in and earthbound states of sanity, could never compose the *Messiah* or *Mrs Dalloway,* and this mad state of genius is, in a proverbial nutshell, why not.

In addition, we cannot overlook the fact that the creation *exists:* Schumann's Cello Concerto in A Minor soars; van Gogh's furored strokes swirl auras around so many stars. Perhaps it is the awe that these rarest works of art inspire that leads the academic discussion of madness step by step into the dangerous and alluring eddy of romanticization. The scholarly treatment of madness may not march in celebration through the streets, but in some ways the disciplined restraint implied by the language of critical theory that emerged over and over again at this conference is at best a façade over just this kind of salutation. At worst it is an example of how distant the ivory tower can be from the reality of human experience. 'No one works better out of anguish at all,' James Baldwin said; 'that's an incredible literary conceit.'

When a terrified psychotic patient nails the doors and windows of her house closed and huddles in a corner for days without food or sleep, believing that she is being hunted by alien agents, it is difficult to characterize her schizophrenia as a 'fragmentation of the capitalist self', as I once heard the illness described at an academic conference. When I watch a friend of mine lose her job, her spouse, and finally her will to live to the relentless claws of a bottomless depression, I cannot take seriously the theoretical classification of those who suffer from mental illness as 'existential radicals'.

My mind churns with example after example of lunacy's cruel

baseness: A woman with postpartum psychosis who repeatedly and viciously attacks her husband because she believes he is trying to kill their baby and spends the first two weeks of her daughter's life in a locked psychiatric ward racked with devastating delusions that her baby is in grave danger. An elderly man so gripped with dementia that he shouts and swings at any person who approaches him, fearing that the aides who change his clothes are trying to molest him and that the daughter he does not recognize is trying to feed him poisoned food. A middle-aged banker who believes he must save the world and secretly hoards his feces in a drawer in a hospital's intensive psychiatric unit. It is certainly possible that, like the good and bad sides of the same coin, whatever predisposes the famously mad artists to mental illness also predisposes them to beauty, artistic vision, or creative drive. But even if it is madness that makes possible extraordinary creation, how much ingenuity and productivity are short-circuited by that same madness? How much potential greatness is lost in insanity's dark corners?

Mental illness, and the suffering it carries with it, can consume a person's whole life. And when it does, there is no room for the most basic pleasures, let alone the loftiest of great creations. For my patients, madness is not a political statement. More important, it is something by which hardly any of my patients would choose to be burdened. For those of us who are fortunate enough to be comparatively sane, it is abhorrent to stand in celebration of Woolf's madness. It did, after all, cost her her life. It is audacious and self-serving of us to celebrate mental illness as rebellious and brave, as productive and ingenious, as the mythical, maniacal muse of our artists and writers. At the end of so many of these stories, we are left with their masterpieces. But the lives behind the stories are riddled with suffering and hospitalization and suicide. The brilliant psychologist and author Kay Redfield Jamison has said that bipolar disorder – an illness from which she herself suffers – 'benefits mankind at the expense of the individual'. Who are we, exactly, to say that it is worth it? Even if madness is at the root of some of the world's great creations, it is hard to imagine that if someone asked each of us to live an entire life of suffering in the service of the arts, we would agree to do so. Even if we might choose such altruism, it's unlikely we would allow anyone else to make that decision for us.

And as fiercely as we hold to this romantic argument of greatness arising from madness, are we sure we have it right? What if the opposite is true in the cases we cite of van Gogh and Schumann and all their sad, mad peers? What if the greatness of these artists existed not because of the madness but in spite of it? Might our mad creators – and the countless other artists who were so afflicted – have blossomed even more fully if not hindered by depression or haunted by psychosis? For Plath and Woolf and Sexton and others who prematurely ended their own lives, we must also consider what further genius might have arisen over the full course of their lost years.

There is no glamour in my patients' lives. For the vast majority of them, their daily existence holds much misery, and no romance. And yet it is comforting to those of us gifted with sanity to believe that there might be some redeeming, glorious, even magical aspect to the deadening, punitive force of madness. There is surely veracity in Woolf's description of her mental illness, but in celebration of the 'lava' of madness and its fantastic by-products it is all too convenient to lose sight of the story's end: a brilliant woman loading her overcoat pockets with stones and stepping into the river Ouse to die.

'I feel certain that I am going mad again', Woolf wrote to her husband in her suicide note. 'I feel we can't go through another of those terrible times. And I shan't recover this time. I begin to hear voices, and I can't concentrate. So I am doing what seems the best thing to do. . . . I can't fight any longer. . . . You see I can't even write this properly. I can't read. . . . Everything has gone from me but the certainty of your goodness.'

In the earliest moment of morning, a mockingbird perches on our neighbor's redbud tree and lets fly trill after trill, fluted note after fluted note. Our bedroom windows have been cracked open all night just enough to let in the mossy chill of spring. In the daytime I find this bird's song to be an enthralling spectacle of flawless copies: now a pewee, now the mewing squawk of a catbird, now the whistle of a wren. I could listen all day. Sometimes I do. But at 4:00 A.M., burrowed beneath an old quilt and half aware that my young children have managed, for nine hours, to sleep soundly without a single 'Mama,' the mockingbird's call grates at me, all painful awakening and incessant noise. If I could throw a pillow out the window and hit my mark, I'd have to say I would.

It's a reminder. The thing stays the same. It's our vantage point that changes. Humanity has a fickle vein in which something can be sometimes loved and sometimes hated. What is it that tilts the balance?

I used to sleep until midday if I could. When I was a teenager, a twenty-year-old even, visiting my grandparents on a school vacation, my grandfather would cackle to see me rise, all rose-cheeked and rumpled. 'Eleven o'clock!' he'd crow. 'Oh, to sleep like that.'

My grandmother, a great bird-watcher, would've been up hours and hours earlier to see what she could see. I wish I'd asked her, before she died, what it was about birds that she loved so much. She was, however, prejudicial in her admiration. She'd tell me a hundred times about tramping through the northern Michigan jack pine forests with her friend Kay to catch a lucky glimpse of a Kirtland's warbler. Then, just as often, she'd disparage 'those horrible starlings', or curse the invasive merganser ducks that infiltrated our Michigan lake.

I call my mother, now that I cannot ask my grandmother for her own answers. 'Didn't Grandma have some reason not to like mockingbirds?'

I ask my mother. No, she says. Not that she can remember. 'Are you sure? I thought they laid eggs in other birds' nests and then their babies grew bigger than the others and took all the food, and . . .' I'm thinking of cowbirds, my mother tells me, which, yes, Grandma loathed. But mockingbirds? Nothing rings a bell.

My grandmother could be ruthless, in the way that nature also can. A cardinal built a nest outside her first-floor window, and I mentioned it to her, delighted. 'If that bird is dumb enough to build its nest that low,' she scoffed, 'it deserves to have its eggs eaten by a snake.' They had a garden and a little orchard at their rural Indiana home, and one Saturday of my childhood I ran to the blueberry bushes only to find a sparrow who had died after it got twisted in the netting around the bushes. 'He shouldn't have tried to eat my berries,' she said. Still, I noticed how tenderly she untangled him from the nylon threads. She held the body in her palm and had me look closely at what we rarely had the chance to see: beak, and wing, and claw.

My brother and I took a garden spade and dug a grave for that sparrow beneath the peach tree, solemnly marking it with . . . what? The pink-white flower from a pea tendril? A fat zucchini blossom? Clover? I can't recall. But for nights after, lying in my twin bed, I'd think not of the dying but of the struggle. How flight turned into entrapment. How little the poor bird must have understood. How the more it moved, the more tangled its feathers would have become.

People who have schizophrenia are more prone to kill themselves in the early stages of the disease than at any other time. The theory is this: A person in his first psychotic break is in a kind of netherworld. He has had years – maybe eighteen, maybe twenty – of sanity. Then the voices come, or the visions, or the paranoia, and he begins to occupy a space in which the symptoms are present but so is his awareness of the stable life that is slipping from his grasp. It is a horrible kind of bridge – the interspace between sanity and brokenness. *Schizo-*, 'to split'. *-Phrenia,* 'mind'. Later – it's awful to say – he likely won't be as aware of what he's lost. Yet in that first grip of madness's net, in that first struggle and the sanity that comes after, he can understand the implications. The full impossibility of escape. *I'm not sure about this existence,* Colin had said to me. *Are you?*

As we prepared him for discharge, Colin said he couldn't promise us that he would continue the medication once at home. And the day he left, I felt unease in the pit of my stomach. I told Colin that I wished him well and reached out to shake his hand. He grasped my hand in both of his and held on, longer than he ought to have. He looked deeply into my eyes, as if he saw something there.

'I wish the best for you, too, Dr Montross,' he said earnestly, with a meditative smile. 'I really do.'

I worried for Colin after his discharge. I worry about many of my patients after they have left the hospital. 'There are two kinds of psychiatrists', wrote Robert I. Simon, himself a forensic psychiatrist. 'Those who have had patients commit suicide and those who will.'

My most memorable patient encounters come from interactions with my schizophrenic patients. They tell me all kinds of things about myself.

'Montross? Like "mantra",' said one, smiling in adoration.

'You will die in your sleep tonight by my hand,' said another. It can be unnerving.

Once, from his jail cell, a man said to me, 'I know you!' I thought perhaps he did. A past psychiatric admission, maybe. Something else. 'We smoked crack together!' he announced triumphantly, as if I had simply forgotten.

Riddled by voices, overcome by delusions, or persecuted by fear, these patients are pressed to take action in the world. And though the results of their actions can be ridiculous, or terrible, there is sometimes an unmistakable urge toward goodness behind their errant behavior. One of my patients bought hundreds of dollars' worth of lighters in an attempt to stop gangs from setting fire to abandoned buildings. Another was brought in by police when, having caught a pigeon whose foot was injured, she held the bird in her lap with a fork and a pair of pliers to try to operate on it.

Because the content of delusions is so frequently religious, my patients have all kinds of ideas, too, about God. They are God, or are sent by God, or are persecuted by him. He has told them to fast, or to take drugs, or to beware of me. When I'm with them in the midst of their torment, I wonder about God more than at any other time in my life. After the writer Annie Dillard read a book about human birth defects, she imagined herself 'hollering at God the compassionate, the all-merciful, WHAT'S with the bird-headed dwarfs?' It's a fair question.

While I was treating Colin in the hospital, I learned a little bit about Amma the Hugging Saint. At first I hadn't even been sure she was real; then, standing in line for coffee at a Providence bakery, I saw a bookmark-size flyer tacked to a community bulletin board. 'Amma: Summer Tour', it read, 'Marlborough, MA. All programs held at the Best Western Royal Plaza Hotel'. An Indian woman beamed in a photograph on the flyer. Her hands were clasped in front of her face, as if she had just seen something that absolutely delighted her. 'Programs include inspirational music, meditation, spiritual discourse, and personal blessings', the flyer read. Beneath the photograph of Amma was a quote attributed to her: 'God is deep within us. He dwells there in pure and innocent love'.

There is plenty of footage of Amma on the Internet, and it turns out that she's been covered by major newspapers. A 2006 movie was made about her, called *Darshan: The Embrace*. In 2010 she received an honorary degree from SUNY Buffalo in recognition of her humanitarian efforts.

Amma was born in southern India. Her father was a poor fisherman.

The *New York Times* reports that Amma 'was said to have been born with a bluish hue to her skin and became an outcast. Her father withdrew her from school in the fourth grade and made her serve as a family slave'. As an explanation of her mission, Amma explains that her childhood meant that she 'had direct experience with the suffering of others. . . . I always wanted to know the cause of misery and thought if sorrow is a truth then there must be a cause and a way out. I realized my purpose is to console, to personally wipe away tears through selfless love, compassion and service'. As a teenager she began hugging strangers on the streets of her village. In the opening minutes of the movie *Darshan,* a teenage Amma is shown with a man whose skin is covered in boils. The voice-over tells us that many of the boils were covered in pus. Young Amma delicately licks one after another after another, then looks into the face of the man with great compassion.

These days her physical contact is limited to hugs, but devotees report that her hugs are life-changing, transformative. Even relative skeptics, such as Jenny Kleeman, a journalist who wrote for the *Guardian* about the experience of hugging Amma, described the encounter as 'the most enjoyable hug I've had from a stranger'.

In Hinduism the concept of *darshan* describes the reciprocal interaction between a deity or guru and his or her followers. The revered person is beheld, and the person who beholds her subsequently receives a blessing. Amma travels the world performing her *darshan* – the hugs – for up to fifty thousand people in a twenty-hour session. According to her followers, Amma has hugged more than 27 million people worldwide. 'She never seems to tire', reports the *Times*. 'Speaking in Malayalam, the language of her native state, Kerala, and translated by her chief disciple, Swami Amritaswarup, she said, "People's happiness is my rest."' A 2006 article in *USA Today* about one of her sessions of *darshan* notes that Amma 'never flinches from the tide of pain and confusion'.

I had initially imagined Colin following Amma through the mountains of the American West on foot, a hiking disciple who followed a guru through rugged terrain by day and pitched a tent with her devotees at night. My image had been one of campfires and drum circles, not of banquet rooms in a string of suburban Best Westerns. Nonetheless, my questions about Colin's experience – and the etiology of his symptoms – remained the same. Does a young man seek Amma the Hugging Saint because he is fragile, susceptible to unconditional acceptance and a persuasive atmosphere? Or is he delusional already and his sense of deep meaning and connection with her is derived wholly from an imbalance of neurotransmitters? Or what if – despite his fragility or illness – he is right after all and she *is* a deity or a saint? There is fervent faith and there is psychiatric hyperreligiosity. Both can be characterized by agonizing self-debasement. Both can bring about ecstatic joy. At what point does a transformation in one's thoughts become something to be treated by medication? When does it become so severe as to impinge upon one's liberty?

I n the *British Journal of Psychiatry,* Yair Bar-El and his colleagues describe Jerusalem syndrome, an acute 'psychotic decompensation' that afflicted 1,200 tourists to the Holy Land from 1980 to 1993. 'On average', the authors write, '100 such tourists are seen annually, 40 of them requiring admission to hospital'. The paper divides the patients into three categories. The first is made up of people who have already been diagnosed with a psychotic illness before traveling to Jerusalem. 'Their motivation in coming to Israel', the authors write, 'is directly related to their mental condition', frequently involving delusions. A subset of these patients 'strongly identify with characters' from the Bible 'or are convinced that they themselves are one of these characters'.

Visitors in the second category lack a psychiatric diagnosis but have what the authors call 'idiosyncratic ideations'. These are groups or individuals with 'unusual ideas' who are 'outside the mainstream of the established churches'. They settle in Jerusalem believing, for instance, that doing so will bring about the resurrection of Christ. They may 'wear distinctive clothing which, according to them, is similar to that worn in the days of Christ'. At some point these patients shift from merely harboring extreme religious beliefs to engaging in behavior that becomes more problematic. Bar-El and his coauthors give the example of a man who set out to preach his message of 'true religion' to the people of Jerusalem and eventually, in the Church of the Holy Sepulcher, 'succumbed to an attack of psychomotor agitation and started shouting at the priests, accusing them of being pagans and barbarians and of worshipping graven images'. Eventually the altercation became physical, and the man began destroying paintings and statues in the church, resulting in his psychiatric evaluation. He was found to have no identifiable mental illness beyond his extreme religious beliefs, even three years after the episode.

It is, however, the third category of tourists afflicted by Jerusalem syndrome that is the most mind-boggling. This category is described as a 'pure' form of the syndrome, because its sufferers have no history of mental illness. These tourists experience an acute psychotic event while in Jerusalem; they recover 'fairly spontaneously, and then, after leaving the country, apparently enjoy normality'. As a result they are considered to be mentally well, but for these isolated episodes. However, what episodes they are!

Tourists with the third subtype of Jerusalem syndrome succumb to a sequence of identifiable stages that are consistent, characteristic, and highly specific.

First, such sufferers exhibit 'anxiety, agitation, nervousness and tension'. They then announce that they wish to split off from their tour group or family and explore Jerusalem on their own. The authors write, 'Tourist guides aware of the Jerusalem syndrome and of the significance of such declarations may at this point [preemptively] refer the tourist . . . for psychiatric evaluation'. They add ominously, 'If unattended, [the following] stages are usually unavoidable'.

People afflicted by Jerusalem syndrome will then demonstrate a 'need to be clean and pure', becoming obsessed with bathing or compulsively cutting their finger- and toenails. Next is my favorite step in the sequence: the 'preparation, often with the aid of hotel bed-linen, of a long, ankle-length, toga-like gown, which is always white'.

Once appropriately clad, the person in question will proceed to 'scream, shout, or sing out loud psalms, verses from the Bible, religious hymns or spirituals'. He or she will then proceed to a holy place within the city and deliver a sermon, which the authors describe as 'usually very confused and based on an unrealistic plea to humankind to adopt a more wholesome, moral, simple way of life'.

The affected person typically returns to normal within five to seven days, feels ashamed about his behavior, and recovers completely. Between 1980 and 1993, the authors report that forty-two cases met all the diagnostic criteria for this third subtype.

Similar syndromes have been reported in Paris and Florence, each with its own odd specificities. Paris syndrome strikes Japanese tourists, sixty-three of whom were hospitalized with the condition between 1988 and 2004, according to a paper in the French psychiatric journal *Nervure*. Apparently the condition was common enough – and severe enough – that the Japanese embassy arranged for a Japanese psychiatrist to assist in treating cases at the Parisian psychiatric institution Hôpital Sainte-Anne. The Canadian philosopher Nadia Halim notes in her paper 'Mad Tourists' that 'Paris holds a "quasi-magical" attraction for many Japanese tourists, being symbolic of all the aspects of European culture that are admired in Japan.' Tourists who fall victim to

Paris syndrome 'arrive in Paris with high, romanticized expectations, sometimes after years of anticipation, . . . unprepared for the reality of the city. The language barrier, the pronounced cultural differences in communication styles and public manners, and the quotidian banalities of contemporary Paris – the ways in which it is like any other 21st-century Western city – induce a profound culture shock' that results in symptoms ranging 'from anxiety attacks accompanied by feelings of "strangeness" and disassociation, to psychomotor issues, outbursts of violence, suicidal ideation and actions, and psychotic delusions'.

In the 1980s Graziella Magherini, an Italian psychiatrist and psychoanalyst, identified a syndrome in Florence in which visitors to the city become emotionally unmoored by their encounters with its art and architecture. Magherini reports on 106 cases from Santa Maria Nuova Hospital over ten years. Symptoms include breathlessness, palpitations, panic attacks, and fainting or collapsing to the floor. Severe cases have involved persecutory delusions and paranoia.

Nadia Halim writes in 'Mad Tourists' that in many of Magherini's case studies 'patients report some sense of disintegration' or feel themselves breaking apart. After becoming transfixed by Caravaggio's *Bacchus,* a fifty-three-year-old man felt 'there was no longer any precise definition' in his life. The *New York Times* reports an event in front of the same painting, in which a man 'collapsed onto the floor of the Uffizi, thrashing about madly. He was carried out on a stretcher, raving and disoriented'.

Also according to the *New York Times,* a twenty-five-year-old woman named Martha 'became "delirious" after standing for a long time before the Fra Angelico paintings in San Marco. She returned to her hotel', the *Times* reports, 'and stood for a long time in a corner, mute and withdrawn.' A twenty-year-old woman was seized by terror in the Uffizi and screamed for help, believing that she felt 'the anguish of breaking into a thousand pieces'. Halim writes that she was 'so agitated she had to be physically restrained'.

A 2009 paper in the *British Medical Journal* describes a seventy-two-year-old artist who went to Florence 'to fulfill a lifelong wish to see the art and culture that so inspired him. He described some works of art as "like seeing old friends".' The Ponte Vecchio apparently had a particular allure for him, being 'the part of Florence he was most eager to visit'. Once he was standing upon it, he had a panic attack, became 'disoriented in time', and became floridly paranoid, believing, among other things, that his hotel room was bugged and that he was being monitored by international airlines. His symptoms resolved in three weeks.

Magherini dubbed the condition Stendhal syndrome after the French author of that name who became overwhelmed as a result of viewing the frescoes in the Church of Santa Croce. Stendhal wrote that as he exited the church, the sight of Brunelleschi's dome on the Florence Cathedral nearly led him to madness. 'I felt a pulsating in my heart', he wrote about the experience. 'Life was draining out of me. I walked with the fear of falling.' He was cured only by sitting down to read the poetry of Ugo Foscolo, who had written about Florence and hence was 'a friendly voice to share my anguish'.

The mere existence of these 'city syndromes', as Nadia Halim dubs them, is controversial. Many voices have weighed in to argue that these episodes are merely exacerbations of preexisting psychiatric disease or the initial onsets of mental illnesses that happen to occur in foreign cities. Still others have chalked up the circumstances to jet lag or some other mundane variety of travel-related disorientation. At this point no one knows.

I didn't meet Colin before he traveled with Amma across the American West. Which came first, the symptoms of his illness or the experience and promise of his transformation? He might have begun to exhibit subtle signs of mental dysregulation before he left to follow Amma, and then the stress and stimuli of travel caused his symptoms to explode. Or he might have been completely healthy before his trip and then gone to the mountains and taken some hallucinogens, at which point his bizarre beliefs and behavior began to emerge and his illness was unmasked. I got to see Colin only when he was already ill, without the benefit of knowing whether holiness, or place, or beauty had anything to do with the mental illness that had derailed him.

One morning a woman named Nancy was admitted to my inpatient service. 'Why do we look alike?' she asked me suspiciously, though she was twice my size and a different race. Before I could answer that I wasn't sure we did, she demanded I recite the Fourth Amendment. I couldn't. 'Will you kindly get the fuck out of my room, then, and send in an American?' she asked. I left and looked it up. Ah, search and seizure. Needing a warrant. Now I know.

Nancy was in filthy clothes, and because she held a paranoid belief about the city's having poisoned the water supply, she had not bathed or brushed her teeth in weeks. I knew from reading the report from her physical exam that she had a fungal infection beneath her breasts where they lay against her abdomen because it had been so long since she had washed herself there.

I treated Nancy for the first two days of her admission, but while she remained hospitalized, my clinical assignment switched and I began covering a different unit. When my schedule shifted back to her unit three weeks later, I saw Nancy's name on the board and remembered our encounter. I was curious about her progress and went out on the ward to talk with her. I scanned the whole unit twice and could not find her. Alarmed, I finally approached the nurse in charge of the unit.

'I can't find a patient. I've looked everywhere,' I announced, flustered.

'Which one?' asked the nurse.

'Nancy,' I replied. 'Nancy, with paranoid schizophrenia.'

The nurse looked at me quizzically. 'She's right there,' she said, and gestured to a well-groomed and neatly dressed woman ten feet away from me in plain view, drinking coffee and reading the *Providence Journal*.

I went over to Nancy. 'Excuse me,' I said. 'I'm Dr Montross, Nancy. We've actually met once before.'

'I'm sorry, Doctor, I don't remember,' Nancy responded, smiling politely at me. 'It's been a bit of a rough patch for me lately. Would you like to sit down?' I did, and we proceeded to have a perfectly lovely conversation about how she was feeling ('Oh, much better, thank you') whether she was having any problems with her medications ('They always make me a little drowsy at first, but that's passing now') and her plans for the future ('My husband's been taking care of our dog, so I'm anxious to get back home to our apartment. He doesn't spoil that dog the way I do').

When I left Nancy, I went to the computer and read sequentially through her progress notes since I'd seen her last. My evaluation was first, documenting how she'd been out of treatment for four years prior to her admission, that she'd also accused the emergency-room physicians of violating her Fourth Amendment rights, and that she'd claimed to be homeless despite living with her husband of twenty years. She had, at the time of her admission, said that she had three children, all of whom had died of AIDS. In fact, her three grown children were alive and well and, according to the nurses, had been in to visit her several times during her hospitalization.

Subsequent physician notes revealed that Nancy had been paranoid and agitated for nearly a week after she was first admitted and that she had refused to shower or eat, convinced that the water and food were poisoned. Eventually the primary psychiatrist who was treating her took her to mental-health court. In certain circumstances, which vary from state to state, a clinician can use the same rationale that provides for hospitalizing a person against her will (danger to self or others or 'grave disability') to make a petition for court-ordered treatment. In cases such as these, which go beyond an initial involuntary hospitalization, a judge may rule that the patient must remain hospitalized, even if she does not wish to do so, and must also take the psychiatric medication she is prescribed.

The judge ruled with the psychiatrist in Nancy's case, and Nancy remained in the hospital and was treated with antipsychotic medication. Relatively quickly her symptoms abated, and she improved.

Taking away someone's autonomy is an uneasy balance. In Nancy's case, with the benefit of hindsight, we now know that it was the right thing to do. As a psychiatrist, I find it immensely rewarding to see a patient delivered from fear. And this trajectory is shared by many patients, because for all the vagaries of psychiatric medications, correctly prescribed antipsychotics frequently *do* treat psychosis in precisely this way.

Our psychiatric diagnoses are not always as clear as we would like or as well defined as we may believe. We can't be sure whether a person feels his life disintegrating because of Caravaggio's puissance or because of jet lag and an underlying predisposition to mental fragility. We must weigh whether a young man has the right to fast and adopt bizarre – potentially dangerous – behaviors if he believes himself to be the devout disciple of a saint. Surely we should tread with extraordinary caution when we infringe upon our patients' freedoms. And yet, as Nancy and many other patients have taught me, that doesn't mean we aren't sometimes obliged to do so.

We all long, at some point, for a profound awakening. We travel with the expectation that the places we see and the encounters we have will transform us. We go to theaters and museums and holy sites in the hope of discovering something that will have a new and permanent resonance in our lives. It's a human hunger. We *want* transformative things and places and people to exist in the world, and we want to be able to tap into their power, to use them to see our lives with a new and greater clarity.

The truth is that these transformations – these awakenings – exist. Their power is experienced in galleries and on mountaintops, in libraries and in temples, at rock concerts, on psychotherapists' couches, and in scientific laboratories. They may be subtle or life-changing, as when the young Alexander Calder, working as a fireman on a ship, reportedly woke from sleep on the deck to a sky that held both a full moon and a dazzling sunrise. The sight inspired him to become an artist.

And yet there is a line beyond which transformation can lead to upheaval. On the other side of the line is illness. Determining the moment at which this line has been crossed is difficult and inexact. As a psychiatrist, I cannot practice in hindsight. I must balance the benefits of early, preventive care with the preservation of my patients' civil liberties and choices. Often I see patients immediately after their illnesses have thrown them deep into the wells of personal devastation. But on rare occasions I see patients just *prior* to when the devastation is set to begin. In those cases, how can I preserve their autonomy up to that mythical line and then jump in to treat them precisely in time to prevent them from wreaking total havoc on their lives?

As an example, I recently treated Monica, an undergraduate honors student who had chosen to film a documentary on homelessness for her senior thesis. She began by forging a connection with a clergy member who helped run a local women's shelter. With the help of that mentor, Monica arranged interviews with shelter residents. However, as the stresses of senior year increased, she began to feel increasingly behind. In order to stay up late to study and finish work for her other courses, Monica began taking pills from a bottle of prescribed amphetamines her roommate had for ADHD. She began sleeping less and studying more. She continued to take the pills to keep up. Soon she was even more deeply impassioned about her documentary project and felt it had the capacity to ignite real social change. Her professors, her friends, even her parents were impressed by her newfound energy and her urgent conviction to do good. Before long she found she did not need the pills to stay awake. She stayed up for days at a time and hardly needed to eat. Determined to get to the 'real' story of the experience of homelessness, she began working without her mentor and accompanied women, and eventually men, to spend nights with them on the street. When she began not returning home at night, her university roommates became concerned and called Monica's parents, who flew in from Texas. Her parents discovered that during the previous two weeks Monica had covered her body with tattoos and had had sex with multiple strangers, all of which she viewed, at the time, as a means of connecting with the people whose plight she was trying to shed light upon. They immediately brought her to the psychiatric hospital. It became clear, as my colleagues and I evaluated and treated Monica, that her fiery enthusiasm for her project had been the harbinger of a manic episode, brought about – or unmasked – by her use of stimulants. Her dedication to her cause had initially seemed so inspiring, like an awakening. Sadly, the awakening turned out to be a part of her illness, and it fueled her self-destruction.

When I met with Monica's distraught parents, her father asked in desperation, over and over, 'Should we have known? When she called us so excited, should we have . . . ? How did we let this . . . ? When should we have known?' If they had known, I reassured them, they would have intervened. But his desperate question was the very one I sometimes ask myself: At what point can we *know* that ecstasy, or singular purpose, or religious fervor has become pathological, if we don't wish to wait until obvious and irreversible damage has been done? Why subject someone to the risks and potential adverse effects of medicine if her precise diagnosis has not yet been determined? The answer is that this anticipatory, proactive treatment is a fundamental and accepted component of every field of medicine.

When a woman feels a lump in her breast, she does not know what it is. It could be a benign, monthly, cyclical swelling, or it could be a malignant tumor that has already widely metastasized, or anything in between. To zero in on a diagnosis, her doctor may first order imaging – mammography or ultrasound, for instance – to attempt to determine what the lump is. If enough ambiguity remains after imaging, more invasive procedures are conducted: needle biopsies, lumpectomies. If those procedures reveal cancerous growth, still further procedures, such as mastectomies and lymph-node dissections, are routinely conducted to determine whether the cancer has spread. Mastectomies are often done on the basis of a cancerous lump that has been removed, regardless of the fact that there are no signs of cancer in the remainder of the breast. Breasts are even removed prophylactically for some healthy, cancer-free women whose genetics put them at high risk of eventually developing the disease. Women whose cancer has been treated, who have had mastectomies, who have undergone chemotherapy and radiation, who have no detectable cancer in their bodies, may for years still be prescribed medications whose risks and significant side effects are tolerated and endured because the medications have been shown to reduce the odds of breast cancer's recurrence.

In medicine we constantly choose between two evils. We eye the balance, and weigh the risks, and make judgment calls, and predict as best we can. Whether our data include tumor markers and pathology results or a collection of mood symptoms and behaviors that indicate a dramatic change, we are trained to be vigilant but not hasty, to be proactive but not rash. Physicians prescribe medicines in order to ward off cancer recurrences and heart attacks and strokes and diabetes without knowing for sure whether these conditions would ever befall our individual patients if we left them untreated.

Similarly, I do not wish to medicate people who are simply joyous, or loving, or energetic, or passionate. Still, I cannot ignore that the stakes are high if I misread mania for ecstasy or psychosis for divine connection. So I trust in my study of symptoms and the diseases they portend. I question my intuition rigorously and routinely, but I rely upon it nonetheless.

For our tenth wedding anniversary, Deborah and I leave our children with a beloved baby-sitter and return to the Vermont inn where we were married. The four-hour drive from our home, which might have been onerous before we had children, is now a blissful chance to catch up and gossip and pontificate. As I look out the window at hills and hills of trees sliding past us, their leaves beginning to break into the colors of flame, I find that I'm thinking about a question the psychiatrist and philosopher M. O'C. Drury posed about Joan of Arc. 'Supposing Robert de Baudricourt had been able to give Joan a stiff dose of phenothiazine instead of the panoply of a knight at arms', Drury asked, imagining that today the saint's holy visions might be treated with an antipsychotic, 'would she have returned in peace to the sheep herding at Domremy?'

'What *about* Joan of Arc?' I ask Deborah, sharing Drury's question with her as she drives. 'I mean, if I saw someone today with her exact story – message from God, mission to overthrow the government, the whole deal – I don't think there is any way I would come to any conclusion *other* than that she was psychiatrically ill. In fact,' I add, 'I think the same can be said for a whole number of saints and martyrs who saw visions, or flagellated themselves, or fasted for prolonged periods of time. If I saw that today . . .' I trail off.

'But if you saw someone with those symptoms today,' Deborah says, 'and they seemed to you to be at risk, or suffering, are you saying you think you'd be wrong to treat them?'

'No,' I say. 'I think I'd be right to treat them. But what does that mean? Does that mean that psychiatry leaves no room for divinity? That we'd medicate a person out of what could otherwise be a transformative and saintly life? That we'd subjugate – or, worse, block – some message from God?'

'Seriously?' Deborah asks.

'What?' I say.

'Seriously? You're worried that you are somehow blocking God's communication to the world? *Now* who's paranoid, or grandiose, or whatever you call it?' It takes me a minute to see that she is not just teasing me, that she is also – as always – very wise. She is pointing out my overly narrow assumptions about the possibilities of divine experience. 'If there is a God – and you know I'm not sure about that,' she continues, 'but if there is, don't you think that how God reaches us today would necessarily look different than it did in the fifteenth century? And that God would find a way to communicate his message that wasn't thwarted by your little pills?'

I start to grin. 'You mean "Big Pharma" can't kill God?'

'Yes,' she says, grinning with me. 'That's exactly what I mean.'

I still wonder what has become of Colin. I think about my fear of him that first night in the ER as he stared at me and then my imagined diagnoses for him from the photo only, both of which pegged him as angry or dangerous. Knowing what I do now about his expansive happiness and joy, I wonder if something about that much openness – that willingness to really look with love at each of us – was somehow, on some deep level, actually unsettling.

I know that my fear is that today Colin is lost somewhere with full-blown psychosis, that his happy delusions have turned to horror, or, worse, that he resumed a spiritual fast that his body eventually could not withstand. Still, I understand the urge to hope that there are people like Colin whose symptoms do not necessarily indicate a debilitating illness but rather a prophetic gift or a deep connectedness to the world.

The romantic interpretation of mental illness gets it wrong. As difficult as it is for me to medicate someone who is doing no harm, who speaks of love and connection and ideas to which we should all aspire, I know, as a physician, that Colin is ill. That too much elation *is* a chimera. But that doesn't mean that those of us who treat patients in the grip of madness do not hear and receive some piece of the messages they give us, even if those messages are rooted in psychosis.

I have stood before Caravaggio's *Taking of the Christ* and felt some piece of myself disintegrating. I have believed something so deeply that I would like to wrap myself in bedsheets and proclaim it from the village square.

Every diagnosis is an act of faith. I trust my own clinical intuition and acumen. That does not mean I do not harbor some uncertainty about whether my judgments are, in the end, the right ones. I *am* certain, however, that in my work I am not trying to diminish my patients' capacity for fervent belief, or creativity, or even eccentricity. Sometimes there is beauty or inspiration in the extraordinary experiences of my patients' lives. More often there is agony. Either way, by the time they come to me, their beliefs or behaviors have begun to threaten their abilities to survive in the world, flawed place that it is.

'This hospital, like every other', Annie Dillard writes, 'is a hole in the universe through which holiness issues in blasts. It blows both ways, in and out of time.' She is writing about a medical hospital, about births and deaths, the comings and goings of life, the beginnings and ends. Yet she specifies – a hospital *like every other*. Like my own. I believe that healing is a kind of holiness. But like any good religion, it leaves me with a fair number of huge and unanswerable questions. The wind blows in. The wind blows out. Above my computer, pinned to a bulletin board next to artwork my children have made for me, a photo of Amma the Hugging Saint beams down at me. Her face is full of abundant and ubiquitous love.

CHAPTER FOUR

I've Hidden All the Knives

I will not let them live for strangers to ill-use,
To die by other hands more merciless than mine.
No; I who gave them life will give them death.
Oh, now no cowardice, no thought how young they are,
How dear they are, how when they first were born –
Not that – I will forget they are my sons
One moment, one short moment – then forever sorrow.

— Euripides, *Medea*

I 've hidden all the knives,' Anna said quietly. She and I had just sat down together in a small interview room on the inpatient psychiatric unit, where Anna had been admitted the night before. I hadn't even had the chance to ask my standard opening question about how it was that she had come to be hospitalized. She looked into her lap as she spoke, and she looked miserable. 'My son is fifteen months old,' she began. 'And lately we'll be in the living room and he'll be watching cartoons and I'll see myself . . .' Her voice grew fainter, then trailed off. I urged her to go on.

'See yourself what?' I asked gently. She glanced up at me, and I could see that her eyes had reddened and filled with tears. Her right thumbnail was digging deeply into her left index finger's nail bed. There was a small, bright spot of blood. She took a deep breath and looked straight into my eyes.

'Drowning him. Or taking a knife,' she said, still quiet but now firm. 'Slitting his throat.' Her gaze stayed on me. My stomach turned; I hoped my face did not betray the way I felt.

Over the years of my training, I have learned the potency of the first words I say to patients after they tell me their central concern. Even the most psychotic patients can retain the human capacity for gauging their listener's response. Often it's a test. A delusional patient may tentatively reveal that the same black van has been behind him in different cities, morning and night, to see whether his fears are dismissed or taken seriously. A pedophile may explicitly describe his fantasies to see how easily you can be shocked, or scared away and led off course. Regardless of the literal content that is disclosed, it seems to me that in such situations the real question these patients are asking is almost always the same: How well can you tolerate my suffering? How well can you sit with the pain?

Nothing about Anna made me feel as if she were trying to shock me. In fact, to the contrary, she seemed as if she had summoned up enough courage to tell me the truth and now was terrified about what I might think of her and of the horrific vision she had conjured. I imagined that if Anna were to tell her family members about these thoughts, they would immediately and appropriately shift their concern to the child. My own thoughts reflexively ran toward him, too. However, it was my job as Anna's psychiatrist to focus on how these visions were affecting *her*. Still, I was better able to do so because Anna was on a locked ward and thus posed no immediate threat to her son.

Her eyes remained on me. I weighed my response. My gut told me that I could empathize with Anna, with how frightening and disturbing it must be for her to have those thoughts. And yet offering that kind of opening might close her down in the event that I was wrong. If I said, as I felt inclined to do, 'That must be very difficult for you,' and in fact part of her shame lay in the fact that she was *not* feeling disturbed by the thoughts, then my assumption would only compound that shame and diminish the likelihood of her telling me how she truly felt.

'What has that been like for you?' I finally asked. She looked at me with incredulity.

'What do you *think* it's been like for me? It's absolute hell! I'm constantly feeling afraid that I might hurt him. And then, I mean, what kind of a mother . . . ?' And here she trailed off once again, tears slipping down her cheeks into the pursed corners of her lips.

'Have you been able to talk with other people about this?' I asked her, sensing from her question that the degree of shame might have prevented her from sharing her fears with anyone who could potentially be a support to her.

'Not in so many words,' she replied. 'I think my mother-in-law is convinced that I didn't really want to be a parent. I'm always asking her to come by and watch the baby, to take him out whenever I'm alone with him. I always make it sound like something urgent has come up, but' – and here she allowed herself a small, self-aware smile – 'there are only so many things I can invent that require me to run an errand by myself or be at home alone. She has to be catching on that something is up. I even try to rotate. Sometimes I call my sister, but she's so busy with her own three kids that I feel guilty. I mean, I can't even handle one – how can I ask her to take care of her family and my baby, too?'

Anna's desperation and shame were unmistakable. Yet I still didn't have a clear picture of what she was experiencing when these images came into her mind. I picked up her pale pink hospital chart from the rolling rack beside my chair and quickly paged through it. When I came to the doctor's notes from Anna's evaluation the night before in the emergency room, I took a moment to read through them.

'This is a thirty-four-year-old married female who self-presents seeking help for what she describes as 'the urge to kill my son'', the emergency psychiatrist's intake form read. 'The patient is also having thoughts of killing herself.'

As Anna gingerly continued to talk with me, she eventually elaborated upon what I had found in the chart, though she did not look at me as she spoke. For the last six or seven days, she said, she'd had visions of drowning or stabbing her son, accompanied by voices telling her to see what it would feel like to hold the child underwater. These voices and visions were now coming many times a day, sometimes even multiple times an hour.

I knew I would meet daily with Anna while she was hospitalized and that I would need many sessions with her to more fully understand what she was going through and in what context these symptoms were occurring. Still, in this first meeting, I went through a relatively standardized set of questions and topics to try to learn more about her: Had she ever been to a psychiatric hospital before? (No.) To her knowledge, did anyone in her family have any kind of mental illness? (There was an uncle who'd been depressed and another one who drank too much.) Was there ever a time that she had felt that drugs or alcohol were a problem for her? (She got pretty drunk a few years ago on New Year's Eve, she said. Did that count, if it was only once? No, I said. Then no, she said.) Eventually, with the basic initial questions covered, I returned to the issue at hand.

'I can hear how upsetting these last days have been for you,' I began. Then, gently, 'How likely do *you* think it is that you might actually hurt your son?'

Anna closed her eyes, then opened them and refocused on the corner of the room beyond my chair, where the gray-painted cinder-block walls joined each other and met the floor.

'I don't want to hurt him,' Anna said, beginning to cry. 'I'm just so afraid I might get worn down and give in.'

'Give in?' I asked.

'To the voices, to that urge.' She paused, but I could tell she had something more to say. She took a few breaths, bit her bottom lip, and looked up at me. 'I'm not the kind of person to commit suicide,' she said. 'I don't want to, and religiously, I believe it's wrong.'

'Okay,' I said, waiting to hear where she would go next.

'And it's not like I've been planning how I would kill myself or anything. It's just . . .' Her crying turned to sobs. 'I don't know how much more of this I can stand.'

Once I finished my initial meeting with Anna, I returned to the nurses' station to write in her chart. Immediately the unit staff circled me and talked over one another: Was I sure she had told me everything? Did I realize she wanted to see how it felt to drown her baby? Did I think she was trying to get attention, or was she really that screwed up? They made their collective opinion clear: They had seen all kinds of patients working on a psych ward, but Anna was dangerous and her symptoms were particularly galling.

Eventually Dawn, the formidable and unflappable nurse in charge of the unit, made her way toward me, and the circle dispersed. Only one day earlier, I had seen Dawn march down the hallway addressing multiple patients' problematic symptoms quickly and effectively without slowing or missing a step. 'Kevin, pull up your pants,' she said to a patient who commonly masturbated in public. 'Susan' – and here she addressed a woman who was admitted time and again for cutting and burning herself – 'by hitting the wall, you're telling us you don't think you're safe to go out on the walk with the rest of the group.' Dawn was a real veteran, and despite my medical degree she clearly outranked me in clinical experience. When she had something to say to me, I listened.

'That Anna freaks me out,' she said quietly, leaning over the desk beside me. 'I hope you're not thinking of sending her back home with her kid. I'd hate to be the one with that hanging over my conscience.'

I hated it, too. But I also knew that it is more common than one might think for mothers to have thoughts of killing their children. A 2008 article in *Comprehensive Psychiatry* revealed that in a study of mothers of children under the age of three, 7 percent of nondepressed mothers had thoughts of harming their children. In the group of mothers suffering from depression, that number shot up to 41 percent. In a sample of mothers whose infants were colicky, 70 percent experienced 'explicit aggressive fantasies' about harming their babies. Twenty-six percent of the mothers reported that during episodes of colic they'd had thoughts of killing their children.

Despite my knowledge that many women have these thoughts and few actually act on them, listening to Anna raised in me a mix of emotions, not the least of which was fear about her eventual day of discharge.

On June 20, 2001, Andrea Yates called the emergency line 911. She told the police that she had killed her five children, aged six months to seven years. When the police arrived at her house, she led them to the bodies of her children, whom she had taken one by one to the bathtub and drowned. Despite years of inpatient and outpatient psychiatric treatment – and indeed an appointment with her psychiatrist to which she had gone with her husband only two days before the murders – Andrea Yates succumbed to a series of delusions about herself and her children. A retrospective 2009 article in the journal *Psychiatric Times* reports, 'Ms Yates experienced both depression and psychosis. She believed that her house was bugged, television cameras were monitoring her home, and that Satan was literally within her. She became convinced that her children were not righteous and would ultimately burn in hell. She believed that she needed to kill her children before [they reached] the age of accountability [in order] to save their souls'. The extent of her delusional belief system was obviously not clear to her psychiatric providers at the time, or to anyone else who might have been able to intervene and thereby save the lives of the five children. How, then, could I possibly reach a point with Anna at which I would feel confident sending her home to be with her son?

Without a scientific test to determine whether Anna might be a danger to her son, I needed to better understand her symptoms, so I could determine a more precise diagnosis and treat her accordingly. I needed to talk in depth with her and with her family members to get a clearer picture of what Anna's life had been like recently. I needed to establish and be a supportive relationship for her. Most important, I needed to determine whether Anna fit the profile of someone who *might* murder her child.

We do not know much about women who kill their children. Forty years ago there was almost nothing on the topic in the scientific literature. In 1969 the American forensic psychiatrist Phillip Resnick conducted the first review of the world's literature on child murder. Resnick scoured reports from 1751 to 1969 and found only 155 published cases. (The small number of historically published cases was not an indicator of the infrequency of the killing of children but more likely a testament to how irregularly such incidents were documented. We now have far more data. In fact, the U.S. Department of Justice estimates that, on average, 256 American children were killed by their mothers every year from 1976 to 1994, or one child every thirty-four hours.)

In an attempt to better understand the motives that could lead a mother to kill her child, Resnick proposed a means of categorizing these cases. He first divided them based upon the age of the child and in doing so designated 24 of the cases as 'neonaticides', or killings of children less than twenty-four hours old. The remainder of the cases, in which the children who died were more than one day old, he called 'filicides'. To further underscore the relational factors that distinguish the two, he writes, 'One is the killing of an unwanted neonate within the first few hours of life. The other is the murder of a child after its role in the family has been more fully established.'

Although Resnick went on to publish a paper the following year that reviewed what was known about murders of newborns, this first seminal paper focused only on the 131 documented filicides. It was called 'Child Murder by Parents: A Psychiatric Review of Filicide', and despite the four decades that have passed since its publication in the *American Journal of Psychiatry,* Resnick's classification by apparent motive – the first taxonomy of any kind for these unthinkable acts – remains highly utilized today.

The article established five categories of filicide: accidental, spouse revenge, unwanted child, acutely psychotic, and altruistic.

Accidental murders of children arise not from homicidal intent but rather from abuse or neglect of a child that inadvertently results in the child's death. A pediatrician colleague shared with me one such case she had recently seen in which a mother became drunk and fell asleep on top of her baby while wearing a down coat. She awoke to find the baby not breathing and without a pulse.

Resnick defined spouse-revenge cases as those in which parents deliberately kill their children in order to make their spouses suffer. The mythic Greek character Medea, who kills her two sons to avenge the infidelity of her husband, is the prototypical example within this category. Resnick found this type of filicide to be the least common, and subsequent research has supported that finding. Nonetheless, this motive is not a simply mythological one and might have been at play in the 2010 case of Theresa Riggi, who admitted to having stabbed to death her eight-year-old twin sons and their five-year-old sister in the midst of a custody battle with the children's father.

Murders of unwanted children are more commonly infanticides, as was the case with Melissa Drexler, the highly publicized American 'Prom Mom' who, in 1997, had concealed her pregnancy, gave birth to a baby in the bathroom at her high-school prom, disposed of the infant in the bathroom trash can, and rejoined her friends on the dance floor. However, this motive was also suspected in the equally high-profile case of Susan Smith, who buckled her one- and three-year-old sons into the backseat of her car and let it roll into a lake, where the boys drowned. Smith first achieved infamy because of the racism implied by the fact that she initially claimed 'a black man' had taken her children in a carjacking. Later she was held in even greater derision when court proceedings revealed that one week prior to the incident Smith's boy-friend had written her a letter saying that he liked Smith but did not believe he was suited to raising children.

Acutely psychotic infanticides occur when parents are hallucinating, delusional, or delirious and act out of the fear or anger brought about by their psychotic symptoms. In these situations, Resnick writes, an emotional impulse 'is translated into a violent action'. A mother in this instance might push her son out the window, believing him to be an agent of Satan who intends to kill her. Alternatively, these crimes may be the result of confused, involuntary actions that occur during sei-zures, as when Resnick tells of an 'epileptic mother who placed her baby on the fire and the kettle in her cradle'. In either scenario these are women whose minds are in the throes of a severely distorted reality.

Finally, and most interestingly, mothers who commit altruistic fili-cide believe that their actions are compassionate and driven by love. They kill in an attempt to alleviate their children's suffering – be it real or imagined, present or future. A range of mothers fall within this cat-egory; for example, the mother of a neurologically devastated child who smothered him to put an end to his unceasing seizures, as well as the fifty-year-old paranoid widow who believed that an imaginary slavery ring was attempting to take her eleven-year-old daughter and so mur-dered her to save her from that fate. In testifying on Andrea Yates's behalf at her jury trial, Resnick applied this category of altruistic fili-cide to Yates. In the midst of Yates's psychosis, Resnick argued, her motivation for the murders was altruistic. Yates believed she was saving her children from a lifetime of hellfire and damnation by killing them before they were of an age to be held accountable for their sinful natures. This classification of altruistic filicide would also include mothers who are planning their own suicides and who kill their children so as not to abandon them, or to save them from the grief of their mothers' deaths. This filicide-suicide subgroup is not insignificant. It represented an enormous 42 percent of the women in Resnick's study population, a finding reinforced by the fact that we know approximately 5 percent of mothers who commit suicide also kill their young children.

My task, therefore, was to try to determine how likely Anna was to fall into one of these categories. In talking more with her over the days of her hospitalization, I was able to rule out certain of Resnick's groups, even as Anna's disturbing visions continued. Her son was not an unwanted child, Anna and her husband had been excited to become pregnant, and she continued to say she found joy and meaning in her identity as a mother. Anna's marriage had its share of marital discord, which had been exacerbated by her husband's inability to understand this sudden shift in his wife's mental health, but there was no evidence of the kind of conflict that would lead her to kill her son out of spousal revenge. The child was not neglected or abused. The family confirmed that he had always been healthy, apart from some mild asthma, and I had seen him toddle around the unit one afternoon during visiting hours, chubby and beaming. More important, as Anna and I began to speak to her family members about her symptoms and treatment, every one of them attested to how well loved and well treated the boy was.

My central question, then, was whether Anna was psychotic and, if so, whether her psychosis could be deeply entrenched enough to have tragic consequences. Were the 'visions and voices' she experienced in fact visual and auditory hallucinations that were commanding her to commit acts of violence against her son? Was she able to stay in touch with reality enough to know she should not harm him? Or, as was true for Andrea Yates, was there some secretly held delusional framework within Anna's mind that had led her to believe that killing her son would somehow be an altruistic act of love and kindness?

Dawn's nursing notes reflected her own continued apprehension: 'Patient reports that son and mother-in-law were here for visiting hours. Patient reports that she had homicidal feelings toward her son. Reports voices were telling her to see what it would feel like to stab him. Reports she couldn't wait for the visit to end. This writer suggested patient tell her mother-in-law not to visit with the son. The patient watched football the rest of the afternoon.'

I sat down and talked with Anna again. 'I'd like to talk some more about exactly what you're seeing and hearing when you have these thoughts,' I told her. She nervously nodded her assent. For the first two days, I had treated Anna's symptoms somewhat as I would have treated a trauma victim's flashbacks. The prevailing psychological theories in trauma treatment historically endorsed repeated and detailed retelling of the trauma story by the victim, with the thought that the repetition would dilute the potency of the experience and eventually bring peace and healing. More recently (due in part to research that was conducted in the aftermath of the September 11 terrorist attacks), we have come to understand that retelling the story in a detailed way may in fact be akin to reexperiencing – and thereby deepening the damaging effect of – the trauma. Because I had understood how distressing it was for Anna to experience these visions and suggestions, I had resisted asking her to go over them with me again in detail. Yet Anna's symptoms had not improved in the slightest, despite the fact that I had been giving her an antipsychotic medication for two days now. I was starting to worry that I was missing something.

'Well,' she began, 'it's almost always the same. I'm doing something normal, like laundry or brushing my teeth, and all of a sudden I see this horrible sequence, like a movie in my mind. I'm hurting my son.

I . . . I . . . I kill him, either with a knife or by holding him underwater. I never see myself in that moment, only his body and what I've done to it. While I see this, there's a voice – almost like a voice-over – saying, "Try it. Try it. Just see what it feels like."'

'Then what happens?' I asked.

'Then I see myself bending over his body, so sad at what I've done.' She grew quiet. 'It's so awful to talk about. It's like I'm a monster.'

'Is there ever anything after that?' I asked.

'Sometimes,' she replied. I stayed silent to allow her to continue. 'Sometimes I see myself in jail because of what I've done.'

'Do you ever actually think that you *are* doing it?' I asked her. 'Are you ever unsure as to whether what you're seeing is happening or whether it's only in your mind?'

'Oh, I know it's in my mind,' Anna replied. 'I'm just so scared that one day my mind will overpower my heart, you know? And that I'll act out this film that has played in my head over and over again.'

'How often does it play?' I asked.

'I don't know.' She paused to think. 'Maybe once an hour. Maybe more. It's been happening less since I've been in here, but when I'm around my son, it's going all the time.'

As Anna was describing this personalized horror film looping endlessly in her mind, I began wondering whether these were true visions and voices in the form of command hallucinations or whether they were in fact obsessive thoughts. The difference is a critical one. Obsessions are involuntary, upsetting, persistent thoughts that cannot be reasoned away. Hallucinations are false sensory perceptions. In other words, was she *imagining* this scenario over and over or was she actually, physically *seeing* it?

This was not an issue of mere semantics; my working diagnosis would dictate Anna's treatment, a course of action that, if I were wrong, could have catastrophic consequences. My two potential categories of diagnosis – psychotic versus obsessive-compulsive – called for opposite forms of treatment. If Anna was indeed having command hallucinations to kill her child, the risk that she could fall into Resnick's category of psychotic filicide was a real one, and she should be kept away from her child in order to keep him safe. If, however, this troubling film in her mind was obsessive and not psychotic, then the treatment would call for her to spend *more* time with her son in increasingly distressing and anxiety-provoking settings. This would allow her to see that she would *not* harm him, no matter how strong her fears of doing so might be.

There were risks associated with either course of action. If I wrongly diagnosed Anna as psychotic and made her visits with her son fewer, further between, and more heavily supervised, I would be reinforcing her belief that she could not safely spend time with him. I would also rob Anna's son of a critical relationship with a mother who was loving, albeit afraid. If, however, I incorrectly diagnosed Anna as obsessive and implemented a treatment plan in which she would spend unsupervised time with her son, I could be placing this much-loved toddler in a position of real peril.

My own daughter is seven weeks old when I first take her to our family's Michigan lake cottage. She is a lovely pudge of a baby with a few soft threads of hair, deep cobalt eyes, and a new smile that thrills me whenever it breaks across her face. The May lake is freezing cold, and Deborah and I are wearing jeans and sweaters. But I (who always leap from the car and run down the dock every time I arrive and lift the clear water to my lips the very last moment right before I leave) am determined to introduce my baby to the lake and it to her.

I put her in shorts and a little shirt, slip my hands beneath her armpits, and dip her tiny toes into the green water. A kind of baptism. Her face grows stern and perplexed, as if to ask, *What is this sudden shock of chill?* She pulls her thick, bowed legs up to her belly. I dip her again, then once more, all the while singing gleeful nonsense to her. Smiling broadly, Deborah snaps pictures. Half a moment later, our baby girl threatens to cry, and I concede, cradling her to me and pulling the base of my sweater up around her diapered bottom, her blanched and dripping legs.

That evening my mother pulls the cover off the old motorboat and we decide to take a sunset ride. I swaddle our baby in a beach towel. As I step into the boat with her in my arms, my father holds tight to my elbow, protective, steadying us until I sit down on the bench seat in the bow. My mother walks the boat out to a depth where we can start it without having the prop dig in the sand. Evening's slant of light turns the lake's surface reflective – a metallic, mirrored gray. If I lean a bit over the boat's edge, my head and shoulders cast a shadow that lets me peer into the water, its clarity giving an unobscured view of the sandy lake bottom with its occasional rock, clamshell, furrowed path left by a freshwater snail.

Eventually my mother clambers aboard, revs the motor, and buzzes us around the lake's periphery. With the engine's hum, our baby sleeps soundly; the warmth of her little body against me seeps across my abdomen – the place where she has so recently been inside. In the big end of the lake, the sun begins to dip beneath the tree line, and my mother cuts the motor. We drift to a stop. The water beneath the boat is more than two hundred feet deep, and so even in brightest daytime it is dark and bottomless-appearing. In this half-light of dusk, the water is impenetrably black.

I stand up in the boat's gently rocking bow to take it all in – the quiet, the soft breeze, the sky beginning to burst into a reckless orange glow. As I do, a flash. No other way to describe it. A sure knowledge that if I were to drop my baby overboard, she would sink like a stone and be gone. Fear rises in me, a heartbeat pounding in my throat as I clutch her to me and sit back down. Still, the uncertainty will not relent. Can I keep this small being safe? Can I hold her tightly enough to thwart the peril just beyond the boat's edge? The world; this holy lake; we parents and grandparents of this child, capable swimmers who would instinctively risk our own lives to save her – suddenly none of it steadies or offers protection. There are only my untrustworthy arms, this fragile infant, and these encircling, fathomless depths.

The image of her falling from me is not a wish or an intent. It is a fear. But the fear is such a terrible one that it feels as though *thinking* it might make it so. Between the thought *(I could drop my baby overboard)* and the rational, instinctive reassurance *(But she is safe, and I would never do that)* must be a sliver of a second. What if, during that split second, some motor impulse were to act on the fearsome thought? Some senseless, wild, physical reflex of obedience – unmanaged by reason or love?

I am not by nature an anxious soul. Beyond a ride or two in careening airplanes or the moments in which I received news of serious diagnoses in loved ones, I have never before felt this degree of unremitting fear that makes me tremble, unable to breathe adequately. Never from just a thought, never without real, justifiable external cause. Never since. Back on land, the moment passes. It never returns with that degree of intensity, but similar scenarios resurrect the fear, even if its return is more muted. On a ferry ride from Vancouver to Nanaimo when our daughter is nearly one, I hold her close to me as we look over the rail at the vast expanse of mountains and sea. My heart skips, and I have to step back five feet, then ten from the railing. A year and a half later: At the height of the London Eye, safely encapsulated in our glassy pod, I hold our six-month-old son snugly in a sling. As the space opens beneath our feet, again the catastrophic – and impossible – flash that I might drop him.

Thinking about Anna, I felt the memories of these thoughts resurface. I remembered the boat's edge, the glint of evening on the black lake, and I remembered having felt the steep pitch of fear. But as I remembered those moments, I felt only reflective. Analytical. Calm and secure. I did not *feel* the fear. I only recalled it.

I wonder whether the difference in these situations between someone like me, who happens to be wired on the less nervous side of things, and someone like Anna, who had told me that she had been an anxious person well before she was a mother, is attributable in large part to the persistence of the fear. I was rattled – deeply, but briefly – by isolated thoughts that I could be responsible for the deaths of my children. Anna's violent thoughts might have been of this exact nature. Worst-case imaginings. Devastating what-ifs. And yet, unlike mine, her mind held fast to what was meant to be fleeting. She was unable to let the images go. She became haunted by the thoughts, reliving not only their content but also the terror they fueled. Anna began to believe that she was bound to carry them out if she were not somehow prevented from doing so.

It was not a coincidence that some of my most anxious moments occurred when I was a new mother. In a blog piece for *Scientific American,* the primatologist Eric Michael Johnson points out that the stress hormone cortisol increases in animals (humans included) during pregnancy and in the postpartum period. This underscores what any parent knows: that new motherhood is a stressful time. But it also means that our bodies are operating at a heightened level of vigilance. Johnson argues that increased anxiety in mothers is evolutionarily beneficial. 'Natural selection', he explains, 'has provided mothers with an early warning system, one that can alert them to danger before others are even aware of the risk.'

Whether it was cortisol, or breast-feeding, or any number of other aspects of my physical and hormonal tumult, there is no question in my mind that I have never felt more like an animal than I did in my early postpartum days. I wanted to comfort my infant daughter so fully that her cry was physically painful to me. The smallest signal of her unease would send me rising from much-needed sleep, hoisting my birth-wounded body out of bed and lifting her to me to nurse. Going to her was arduous, but it was nothing compared to the discomfort I felt from her small cry.

The eeriest and most powerful example of primitive postpartum instincts I have ever observed came from Deborah, a mere eight hours after she delivered our son. Worn out from nineteen hours of labor without a wink of sleep, Deborah was finally sleeping soundly in the hospital bed. I was napping fitfully on an awkward recliner beside her when her voice awakened me.

'Christine!' she called urgently. Still primed from the excitement and fear and helplessness of Deborah's labor, I felt a surge of adrenaline rush through my body. I leaped up to her, catastrophizing. Was she bleeding? Was she in pain? Was she safe? 'That's our son,' she said.

'What?' I asked, confused. Our baby boy had been taken to the nursery for routine testing more than an hour earlier. I had no idea what she meant.

'That's him. He's crying. Can you go to him?' Faintly, above the hum of the fan in our window, I heard a baby's cry.

'Sweetheart,' I said, 'get some sleep. There are a million babies on this floor. Half of them are in the nursery. I'm sure it's not our baby.'

And here she grew more urgent – angry, even. 'It's *our son,*' she insisted. Her tired eyes brimmed with tears. She could not yet get out of bed as her body recovered from the delivery. '*Go* to him.' As any non-birthing parent will likely understand, when my partner had endured hours of pain and the associated rigors of childbirth to bring us a child, I would have been inclined to do anything she asked of me. Still, as I padded down the long hallway to the nursery, I thought that this request – and the prospect that Deborah had identified the distant cry as our child's – was ridiculous. After all, our son had cried for a minute at most when he was born. In the subsequent hours in which we held him, wept over him, kissed every centimeter of his perfect form, we had heard nothing more from him than sleepy snuffles.

As I approached the nursery, the cry grew louder but still, to my ear, no less indistinct. I knocked on the door and entered, only to find a swaying nurse shushing our wailing son, who was protesting mightily after his heel had been pricked for a bilirubin test.

I took him from the nurse, swaddled him, and sang to him, and he settled. I wheeled his little plastic bassinet over to our room, where Deborah had fallen back asleep. I held our boy and sat down on her bedside, nudging her awake.

'You won't believe this!' I crowed. 'It *was* our son crying!'

She looked at me with incredulity. 'That's what I *told* you,' she said, reaching out to pull our baby toward her, and then, with him in the crook of her arm, sighed back into sleep.

If Anna's thoughts were true obsessions, she was unlikely to harm her son. However, like many psychiatric symptoms, the manifestations of anxiety run a broad spectrum. And one of the things we *do* understand about mothers who kill their children is that before the murders they are often subjected to enormous amounts of stress.

According to Eric Michael Johnson, this effect may be demonstrated in part in nonhuman primates. He cites research by Dario Maestripieri on macaque monkeys. Maestripieri has shown that the increased cortisol levels in pregnancy are 'directly related to protective behaviors that keep a mother's infant from harm', like when I rose from sleep to feed our hungry daughter or when Deborah sent me off to rescue our son from his blood test. Mothers who are vigilant about their infants' risks and needs are more apt to have offspring that survive, thereby promoting this alertness via natural selection.

However, just as too little maternal cortisol might leave an infant in peril, too *much* maternal cortisol – brought about by prolonged periods of stress – carries with it its own dangers. Maestripieri explains, 'A large body of evidence indicates that extremely high or chronically elevated cortisol levels due to stress can impair maternal motivation and result in maladaptive parenting behavior'. That is, mothers under too much strain may have difficulty as parents. Among Maestripieri's macaques, mothers were sometimes noted to abuse their infants. Those episodes of abuse frequently followed periods of maternal social stress.

In her enthralling book *Mother Nature,* the anthropologist Sarah Blaffer Hrdy meticulously demonstrates that in many species – including humans – mothers kill their children much more routinely than we might imagine. Blaffer Hrdy suggests that animal mothers may eliminate their offspring in direct response to biological and social circumstances. There is, she writes, plentiful biological evidence that mother 'beetles, spiders, fish, birds, mice, ground squirrels, prairie dogs, wolves, bears, lions, tigers, hippopotami, and wild dogs [in] a range of conditions . . . cull their litters and abandon or cannibalize young'.

We may be able to follow – and perhaps even accept – the grim logic by which a mother bird allows an older sibling to nudge a weaker, younger fledgling out of the nest to eliminate competition for food or by which a California mouse kills its pups if it finds itself without a mate to help raise them. Still, even if we accept the logic of survival in those examples, it is difficult if not impossible for most of us to consider human mothers as capable of any similar action. And yet they are.

In his piece for *Scientific American,* Eric Michael Johnson raises this question: Since humans can consciously decide between right and wrong and can 'design political systems that protect the least among us', shouldn't humans be better at protecting our children from maternal infanticide than, for example, 'our distant monkey cousins'?

'The answer to this couldn't be more clear', Johnson writes. In fact, 'humans *are* very different [from our monkey cousins]. . . . We're much worse'. Blaffer Hrdy concurs. As it turns out, our human infanticidal actions are not unique among animals, but they *are* unique among primates. Infanticide 'is widely documented among primates, both human and nonhuman', she writes in *Mother Nature*. 'But in other primates, the killer is almost always an unrelated individual, never the mother. Even when nonhuman primate females are implicated in infanticide, mothers don't harm their *own* infants, they kill someone else's. Only under the direst circumstances does a mother cease to care for her infant or actually abandon it. . . . It is not that unusual for a mother monkey to treat her baby roughly, to briefly drag it, or even punish it with a slap or threaten it with a toothy grimace – especially when she is trying to wean. But no wild monkey or ape mother has ever been observed to deliberately harm her own baby.'

Though Blaffer Hrdy is talking about nonhuman primates, it is not hard to imagine the 'direst circumstances' that might face human mothers, leading them to abandon or harm their children. A study published in the *American Journal of Psychiatry* that analyzed infanticide in seventeen countries emphasizes the contribution of stressful psychosocial factors. The study found an unambiguous 'pattern of powerlessness, poverty, and alienation in the lives of the women' who had killed their children.

'Because killing one's own infant is so abhorrent to us', Blaffer Hrdy writes, 'there is a tendency to compartmentalize the mother's actions . . . to consider her behavior in isolation from her circumstances, even though they are functionally related'.

The laws in America regarding infanticide reflect this isolated abhorrence. England and at least twenty-one countries worldwide grant leniency to mothers who can demonstrate that they killed their children during a postpartum mental disturbance. These laws, based upon Britain's Infanticide Act of 1922, adopt the premise that a woman who has committed infanticide may have done so because 'the balance of her mind [was] disturbed by reason of her not having fully recovered from the effect of giving birth'. The result of this interpretation is that the maximum charge these women can face is not murder but rather manslaughter. The definition of 'infanticide' varies from one country to the next, but in New Zealand the law applies to the murder of children who are as old as ten. America, in contrast, has no federal or state laws that specifically apply to infanticide. Not only may these women be tried for murder, but, as was the case for Andrea Yates, the prosecution may seek the death penalty.

Psychiatrists already know that intense stress increases a new mother's risk for postpartum mood disorders. And social scientists have repeatedly demonstrated that increased parental stress is a risk factor for child abuse and neglect. Stress has also, in various forms, been correlated with a mother's risk of killing her children.

Twenty-five-year-old Lashanda Armstrong had her own share of maternal stress when she drove her van into the frigid Hudson River in 2011, killing herself and three of her four children, ages five, two, and eleven months. The fourth child, her ten-year-old son, who was born when Lashanda was only fifteen, managed to slip out the van door and swim to safety. Though Armstrong was universally described by family and friends as a concerned and highly devoted mother, news reports revealed she was struggling amid difficult life circumstances. A supervisor at her children's day care reported that Armstrong had recently described feeling 'so alone'.

'She's a single parent. She takes great care of her kids, goes to school and works,' said the supervisor. 'She really needed a helping hand.' Armstrong's son had revealed to a teacher that his mother and stepfather, Jean Pierre, were fighting frequently due to Pierre's alleged infidelities. Armstrong was apparently trying to obtain a court order so that he could not have contact with the children. The last time she had left their two-year-old in his care overnight, the child was found by police wandering a city street, barefoot, in a wet sweat suit. The night that Armstrong drove her children into the river, her family had contacted police, fearing that Armstrong and Pierre were 'tussling'. The police reported that the couple had previously had episodes of domestic problems and that an order of protection had been issued – and subsequently violated by Pierre – in the hours immediately prior to the tragedy. *Direst circumstances.*

The forensic psychologist Geoffrey R. McKee created a 'Maternal Filicide Risk Matrix' in an attempt to help clinicians further assess a mother's risk of killing her child. The matrix identifies sources of maternal stress that might combine to make a mother vulnerable to thoughts of child harm. Notably, the presence of a psychiatric disorder is only one of many risk factors. Other potential risk factors that exacerbate the mother's risk of filicide include the following:

teenage motherhood
below-average IQ
less than a twelfth-grade education
no prenatal care
history of trauma (including physical and sexual abuse as well as
    childhood loss of her own mother)
denial of pregnancy
negative attitude toward pregnancy
unassisted birth
nonhospital delivery
difficult birth
absent, abusive, mentally ill, addicted parents during her own
    childhood
violence in partnership

substance abuse in partner
divorce
single parenthood
financial instability
unemployment
relocations
low socioeconomic status
having two or more children if under age seventeen
many children in her care
child difficult to care for
lack of sleep

There is no shortage of anecdotes that highlight the danger in this perfect storm of stressors. Andrea Yates is surely the best-known example. In addition to her documented history of postpartum psychosis, she had for a time lived with her husband, Rusty, and their four children in a 360-square-foot bus. The family had moved into a house by the time Yates delivered her fifth child, but she was still expected to homeschool the older four in the bus while simultaneously caring for her newborn daughter. She had had a string of psychiatric hospitalizations from 1999 to 2001 and an overdose attempt in 1999 after she disclosed a thought of stabbing one of her children. During a period of inpatient hospitalization, she had been so profoundly impaired and unable to care for herself that she had to be spoon-fed.

I used McKee's matrix as a guide in thinking about Anna and the potential risk she posed to her son. Anna was not a teenager, and she had graduated from high school. She was married, though she painted her husband in a less-than-supportive light. Still, there was no evidence of domestic violence or substance abuse in the home. Anna had referenced help from her mother-in-law and sister, though she felt guilty about turning to them for assistance too frequently. She and her husband had stable finances and employment. She had looked forward to the pregnancy and continued to express sincere desire to be a mother – a good mother – to her son.

I understood the immense importance of diagnosing Anna correctly and remained aware that a diagnostic misstep could have disastrous consequences. Still, I was feeling increasingly confident that Anna's symptoms had certain traits that designated them as more obsessive than psychotic. First and foremost, as distressed and fearful as Anna was, she was not out of touch with reality. Over the course of our discussions, she was consistently able to realize that these thoughts were *fears* and not plans. In addition, Anna's responses to the thoughts were characteristic of someone with an anxiety disorder like obsessive-compulsive disorder, rather than a primary psychotic disorder. She tried to avoid the thoughts, and she tried to avoid the situations that brought about the thoughts. Therefore, when Dawn suggested that Anna tell her mother-in-law not to bring the baby in for visits anymore, Anna was relieved and in utter agreement. Finally, and more important, Anna's 'visions' were ego-dystonic – that is, they were repugnant to her and to how she perceived herself. She was deeply and constantly troubled by the thoughts of harming her son, as opposed to someone like Andrea Yates who might have found comfort in a delusional plan that would grant her children eternal salvation. Anna's visions of bending over her son's lifeless body 'so sad at what I've done' and of herself in jail had the feel of compensatory rituals. In the same way that a germophobe might prevent the feared infection by repeatedly washing his hands or following a ritualized pattern of cleaning, Anna seemed to be preventing herself from acting on her intrusive thoughts of harming her son by adding her own punitive epilogue to the horrifying film.

After consultation with colleagues and supervisors and multiple discussions with Anna, I began a gradually escalating course of exposure therapy with her in which she would visit with (or 'be exposed to') her son and then we would meet to discuss the thoughts and feelings she had experienced during her time with him.

I wrote orders for Anna to have structured visits with her son, first on the unit, then leaving the unit with her husband and her son for a few hours at a time, and eventually spending time at home with her son, by herself. At each stage Anna reported increased anxiety, a response that was consistent with an obsessive anxiety disorder. 'The patient reports that intrusive thoughts were exacerbated yesterday during visit with son and husband', my treatment notes read. 'This was very distressing to her.' I make an additional note about her appearance during our meeting: 'The patient is slightly disheveled and nervous-appearing, but cooperative. She taps her fingernails together and on the table. Her hands are tremulous.' As her visits with her son increase in duration and in independence, I note that Anna 'is having an appropriate increase in anxiety level with continued exposure to her son and approaching discharge'. Meanwhile, Dawn's nursing notes indicate that she remains dubious.

'The patient returned from a four-hour pass', she writes. 'Reports that it went fair. Stated "I was with the baby for a half hour and had thoughts of stabbing him." MD still plans to have patient spend time with baby alone despite these ongoing thoughts.'

There was a part of me that felt exactly the way Dawn did. I, too, feared that encouraging Anna to be alone with her son was too dangerous, that the stakes were too high and that I should err on the side of caution. And yet I also felt that in these moments I needed to internalize the very message I was trying to help Anna believe in and hold: that far more women have thoughts of killing their children than actually do; that fearing something does not make it happen; that we have, since Phil Resnick's landmark study in 1969, begun to understand more and more about the women who *do* kill their children so that we can use clinical evidence to help us know those families who are more at risk and those who are less so.

On the twentieth day of her hospitalization, Anna was home alone with her son on a four-hour pass when he had an asthma attack.

'I went right into mom mode,' she said to me on her return, recounting the incident. 'He couldn't breathe and was gasping, and I just grabbed the nebulizer like it was second nature, hooked up the albuterol, and gave him a treatment.' She smiled. 'It felt so great to help him like that.'

One day later Anna was discharged from the hospital with plans to continue treatment on an outpatient basis for obsessive-compulsive disorder. Even after Anna's three inpatient weeks of daily observation and treatment, and her noticeable improvement, I wasn't 100 percent sure of my diagnosis.

Defining the maladies that plague psychiatric patients is an interpretive science. Visions and voices and fear and despair cannot be captured by CT scan or measured in the amplitude of ECG waves. Try as we might, we simply cannot predict which of our patients will kill themselves, which will murder their children, and which will leave the hospital healed, never to return. The reliable portraits and profiles we do have of patients who commit horrific acts are too often, like that of Andrea Yates, available to us only in retrospect, after terrible and irreversible damage has already been done.

With that hindsight, however, we are able to begin to build a framework of understanding as to the symptoms and circumstances that lead women to kill their children. As the field of research begun by Dr Resnick continues to deepen and expand, the act of filicide may remain unthinkable, but it can be less *incomprehensible* to those of us who see or hear about it. If we continue to respond to the idea of child murder by mothers with disgust and scorn for the woman who commits the crime, as we so consistently do, we discourage all mothers – even those who would never harm their children – from feeling safe enough to seek help from the terrifying thoughts that plague them. We cannot prevent all instances of filicide, but if women felt that their disclosure of filicidal thoughts might be met with sympathy and support rather than repulsion and shame, we might have an opportunity to help certain mothers to think more clearly, or to imagine another, better way out.

I never saw Anna again after her discharge. I took solace in the fact that I also never saw her in the headlines. Maybe that meant that my diagnosis of her was right. In any case, the discomfort I felt watching her leave the hospital with her suitcase, her husband, and her son has stayed with me. And yet I had to trust that the child would be safe. It was an awful, uncertain feeling. It somehow seemed right, though, given the fact that it was the exact uncertainty I had asked Anna to trust in and bear.

CHAPTER FIVE

Dancing Plagues and Double Impostors

The mind has great influence over the body, and
maladies often have their origin there.

– Molière

I n my second year of residency training, I spent a month working the overnight shift in the freestanding psychiatric hospital where I am now an attending physician. In theory, my main responsibility during this time was to evaluate people who came to the ER overnight. If they needed inpatient treatment, I would admit them. If not, I would send them off with a list of resources I hoped would be helpful: names of outpatient therapists or psychiatrists, instructions for how to become wait-listed for a day hospital program, addresses and times for local AA or NA meetings.

Some of these decisions were obvious. I admitted a man so paranoid that he had not eaten for days, afraid that he was being poisoned. An alcoholic woman who had no desire to stop drinking had been dragged in by her desperate daughter. With no legal right to hold her against her will, I let her go. Many decisions were not so clear-cut. A woman who had made a suicidal comment to a friend now swore that it was hyperbole. Was she telling me the truth, and would she be safe to leave? Or was she genuinely suicidal but denying it because she didn't want to be hospitalized? A man who routinely claimed he was hearing command hallucinations to inject rubbing alcohol into his veins requested admission at the end of every month, when his assistance checks had run out. At the first of the next month, like clockwork, he would sign himself out of the hospital, stating that his voices had miraculously abated.

In reality, my responsibilities extended far beyond being the gatekeeper of psychiatric admissions. Because this was a freestanding psychiatric hospital and therefore most of the patients were otherwise medically well, I was the only doctor in the hospital overnight. This meant that I was also responsible for any medical issue that might arise on the hospital wards. Frequently I was paged for minor requests: a patient with a headache wanted some paracetamol, or a smoker was in desperate need of a nicotine patch. Sometimes I was called to evaluate a patient with chest pain or to see someone who had taken a fall. Occasionally there were true medical emergencies. When the patients' medical needs were beyond the basic level of care that our psychiatric hospital could provide, they had to be sent out to a medical hospital's emergency room to be treated.

When assessing a patient who needs medical care, different doctors have different thresholds of discomfort, different hierarchies of decision making. I think of it as something like a pain threshold. My own ability to tolerate physical pain is high, a lesson I learned after enduring hours upon hours of labor without medication before our daughter was born. Yet I am also risk-averse, and I err on the side of caution when it comes to patient care. I have colleagues who pride themselves on sending only the very sickest patients out for medical treatment or on admitting only those psychiatric patients who are clearly at the most severe and imminent risk. They joke of being impenetrable 'walls' in the emergency room. They hold it as a point of honor that they do not waste ER doctors' time with psychiatric patients who will surely sleep off their elevated blood-alcohol levels or whose acute chest pain is almost certainly a ploy for narcotics.

I don't want to waste the time of my colleagues in emergency rooms either, but my threshold for sending patients from the psychiatric hospital to the medical hospital is low. This doesn't bother me. I see it as recognizing my own limitations. And probably it's also partially driven by the CYA, as in 'cover your ass', school of medicine. CYA, as a philosophy, is passed down from doctors to medical students in the earliest days of medical training as a kind of inoculation against medical malpractice. It is, of course, an overtly crass and overly simplistic approach, and there are those who would disparage acting to CYA as practicing defensive – rather than clinically indicated – medicine. Nonetheless, I think the gist turns out to be a good gut check: If this ends up being something serious, could people reviewing the chart determine that I should have sent this patient out for medical evaluation? Could I reasonably be expected to have acted differently in my practice by other doctors – or by a court of law?

Sometimes when I send a patient out because I suspect he needs medical attention, I am right, and sometimes I am wrong. Once I was working on the most acute unit of the psychiatric hospital, a ward reserved for patients who were floridly psychotic, or violent, or actively trying to harm themselves. A man who was being treated for opiate dependence was sent to my unit from one of the hospital's general-treatment wards because he had become increasingly psychotic and difficult to manage.

When he arrived on the unit, the patient spoke mumbled nonsense and required constant intervention to keep him from mistakenly wandering into other patients' rooms. When I could understand what he was saying, he was describing women in bikinis looking in his second-story window and men with guns after him about a card game. I suspected he was delirious and sent him to a medical hospital. Delirium can mimic psychosis, with its visions and voices and false beliefs, but it arises from states of medical disequilibrium, like infections or electrolyte abnormalities. In the medical hospital, my patient's blood was found to have precipitously low sodium levels, which had led him into a hallucination-plagued stupor. Had I not sent him out for his sodium to be repleted, he could easily have died.

One week later a homeless patient who had been hospitalized because he was suicidal complained of excruciating foot pain. I pulled off his sock to see a warm, red, and swollen foot. When I pressed my thumb into his ankle, the patient howled, and a deep indentation remained in his flesh where my thumb had been. He had a history of severe infections. I feared he had a cellulitis – a spreading bacterial infection – which could rapidly advance. I sent him to the hospital for what I imagined would be imaging and medication, possibly even admission to the medical hospital for intravenous antibiotics. Four short hours later, the patient was back without even so much as a Band-Aid. His foot, inexplicably, looked better. The somewhat brusque note sent back to me from the emergency physician cited no signs of infection, said the patient had required no treatment, and recommended paracetamol and Epsom-salt soaks should the patient complain of any discomfort. The symptoms never returned. To this day I have no idea what caused his foot's swelling to appear, cause pain, and then recede. The etiology clearly was not the dangerous infection I had thought it to be.

For emergencies, the psychiatric hospital was equipped with a hospital-wide buzzer system. Staff members in every unit had easy access to a blue button and a red button. Pushing either button activated an alarm and illuminated corresponding red or blue lights on numbered panels positioned throughout the hospital. A red light indicated a psychiatric emergency – most frequently a patient who was becoming violent – in which case additional staff members from every unit in the hospital would come to provide extra help. All the staff members in the hospital had been trained as to how to respond to a psychiatric emergency when a patient became violent. My job in those scenarios was to talk with the patient as best I could to try to calm him and to order medications if they were needed. In the event that the situation escalated, requiring staff members to intervene physically, I was to stay out of the way.

However, when the buzzer sounded and the corresponding light flashed blue, it was to notify me of a medical emergency in the hospital. In a medical emergency, though nurses and others were available to help me, I was clearly in charge.

Some psychiatric residents were more gung ho about opportunities to provide medical care than others – those who narrowly chose to specialize in psychiatry over surgery, for instance, or those who had seriously contemplated becoming internists or emergency physicians. I did not fall into these categories. My decision to go to medical school in the first place had been in order to become a psychiatrist. Although to keep myself sane while learning about pulmonary physiology and renal pathology, I stayed open to falling in love with another field of medicine, I never seriously wavered. I felt at home during my rotations with attending psychiatrists, and the knowledge I had to accumulate was more innate to me. No matter how much I studied, the territory of the kidney and lung and heart remained opaque. Their ion exchanges, their functional equations, their vectors, and their voltage-gated ion channels – I could memorize these mechanisms and pass exams to demonstrate that I had done so. But it would be false to say I ever really *understood*.

I could look at an ECG, its needle-traced line on a page, all waves and milliseconds and axes. But it took a kind of faith, I found, to see in that line the aberrant cardiac rhythm that had prevented my grandfather from climbing the stairs to his favorite restaurant. Medicine asks you to believe that an exact equation can explain why an asthmatic six-year-old who lives in a cockroach-infested apartment crosses the threshold from shortness of breath to a prolonged and catastrophic lack of oxygen. You have to live by that math while looking at her in the pediatric ICU, to trust that equation to somehow make sense of her devastated brain no longer able to generate speech, or movement, or comprehension.

In medicine these precise calculations were sacred texts held within a kind of temple that professed to show – exactly – the how and why of sickness, and death, and dying. I found myself a faithless skeptic, disillusioned by the restricted scope and the persistent fight against ambiguity. I could not worship at those tidy altars. Which is not to say that psychiatry is devoid of science. There are those who make this argument, but they are clearly wrong. Nonetheless, our knowledge of the brain is limited, and our knowledge of the *mind* even more so. I found psychiatry's lack of certainty frustrating, yes, but also liberating, and true. There is no satisfying explanation for an eighteen-year-old's first psychotic break; try as we might, there is no way to make sense of it. Perhaps ten or twenty or fifty years down the road, schizophrenia's origins will be made plain. Even so, I expect that knowledge will do nothing to diminish the incomprehension that overcomes me as I try to understand what brings about the fracture of a young man's mind.

So for some of my colleagues and friends, a blue buzzer on an overnight shift was a call to arms and a welcome chance to dive back into medicine's fray. For me it caused a surge of anxiety – would I accurately gauge what was happening? Would I know what to do?

Some residents' entire month of overnights went by without a single blue buzzer. Midway through my August assignment, I had three, one night after the next after the next. The first night a woman who had come in after an overdose suddenly fell down on the unit and was unresponsive. The second night a man had a heart attack. Both times, despite my nerves, I administered medicines and oxygen and sent the patients out by rescue to be treated at medical hospitals – all the correct courses of action. By the third night, even when the trickle of patients into the psychiatric ER slowed and I was able to lie down in the call room to try to catch an hour or so of sleep before the next patient arrived, I couldn't get my mind to settle. I kept waking, staring at the blue buzzer, expecting it to sound.

Eventually it did. I leaped up, grabbed my stethoscope, and ran, cursing what seemed to be my unending bad luck. The psych-ER staff had already sympathetically designated me as a 'black cloud', a hospital term for a young doctor on whose shifts a disproportionate number of bad things occur. I reached the unit that had sounded the buzzer, and the head nurse met me at the door. 'It's Phyllis M.,' she said. 'Do you know her?' I didn't. 'She's here in the Quiet Room.' The Quiet Room was a euphemistically named area of isolation. It was empty. There was no way for patients to hurt themselves or anyone else when they were there. There were strict rules as to how long a patient could be isolated, and the staff worked hard to be sure the patients were there only if – and for as long as – absolutely necessary. Often, patients could be walked calmly there, the door could be left open, and after ten or fifteen minutes they'd be ready to leave again. Rarely, patients had to stay in the locked room for an hour or more; even then they were constantly monitored through a window and evaluated repeatedly in person by the doctor on call. Though many patients have described horrifying experiences with restraint and seclusion in psychiatric hospitals (a particularly searing firsthand description is in Elyn Saks's remarkable memoir of her schizophrenia, *The Center Cannot Hold*), the hospital in which I was working that night takes every measure to use seclusion only when essential and to employ it humanely and safely when it is used. The nurse explained to me how Phyllis had ended up there.

'She's a forty-two-year-old with PTSD, terrible trauma history, comes in from time to time with bad flashbacks. She had an upsetting visit from her mother this evening. Then she kept asking us for Ativan for sleep. When we wouldn't give it to her, she started rocking, pacing, said she didn't think she could be safe out on the unit. We got her to settle down and walk herself to the QR, but then this.'

The nurse gestured down onto the floor of the Quiet Room, where other staff members were kneeling beside Phyllis, whose whole body was convulsing violently. Her head was arched stiffly to one side. As her body shook, her head inadvertently beat against the floor. Her eyes had rolled upward, and a guttural moan was coming from her wincing mouth. She was having a seizure.

A staff member had already stuffed a pillow beneath Phyllis's banging head to prevent her from giving herself contusions or, worse, a concussion.

My own heart pounded while I directed the staff as to how to manage Phyllis's seizure. 'Let's get her on her side,' I said, in an attempt to keep her airway from being obstructed by her tongue and to prevent her from choking on her saliva. 'I'd like to check a pulse ox and a finger stick, please. And let's get some oxygen going.' The mental-health workers began to roll Phyllis to her side, and a nurse scurried to the med room for the equipment we needed and a tank of oxygen. She was back in less than a minute, calling out readings from the monitors and cradling Phyllis's flailing head to wrap the clear plastic oxygen tubing around her ears and into her nostrils. Her blood glucose was normal. She was oxygenating fine. For the time being, there was nothing more to be done.

Seizures require doctors to act counter to their natures. Generally doctors tend to be action-oriented problem solvers. Don't just stand there, do something! The medical maxim of initial seizure treatment is antithetical to this impulse: *Don't just do something, stand there.* Unless a seizure lasts more than five minutes, the course of action in seizure treatment is simply to wait it out. A seizure that lasts more than five minutes may not remit – a dangerous condition called status epilepticus. Without intervention a patient in status epilepticus risks damage to her brain and other organs. Yet prior to that mark, the prescribed course of action is to wait and see. When someone is moaning and convulsing in front of you, five minutes is a long time. Imagine it. Watch the clock.

'Staff was in here with her when she started,' the nurse said, 'so we know exactly how long it's been.'

The mental-health worker who had been watching Phyllis when she began to seize looked down at his watch. 'Three minutes and fifteen seconds,' he said.

That sounded right, since they had hit the buzzer immediately and I'd had time to run from one end of the hospital to the other and be briefed by the nurse. I was paging through Phyllis's chart to look for evidence of a preexisting seizure disorder, or else for medical etiologies or lab abnormalities that might explain why she was seizing. For starters, a huge percentage of our psychiatric medications have the capacity to lower the seizure threshold in a person taking them. This means that patients on certain psych meds are more susceptible to having seizures than they otherwise would be. Phyllis was on several medications that could theoretically be culprits. Other patients are particularly at risk of seizures when withdrawing from alcohol or tranquilizers, but Phyllis had been closely monitored over the five days since her admission and had shown no signs of withdrawal. She'd never had a traumatic brain injury or a stroke that might have predisposed her to seize. Nothing in her medical history stood out. Phyllis continued to groan and convulse. It had been four minutes.

I flipped to the psychiatric section of her chart, and on the third page, buried in a paragraph about prior medication trials, was a sentence that read, 'The patient has a known history of pseudoseizures.'

'Pseudoseizures?' I asked the nurse.

'Oh, yeah,' she said. 'I'm so sorry. I forgot you didn't know her. She pulls this kind of stunt every now and again, but of course we never know if one of them is going to turn out to be real.'

There was judgment in the nurse's characterization of Phyllis as pulling a 'stunt', but there was also wisdom in her assessment of the ambiguity of the situation. Pseudoseizures – more accurately referred to as psychogenic nonepileptic seizures – are, as their name indicates, seizures whose origins are psychological rather than neurological. The idea is a mind-boggling one. The body behaves exactly as it would if the brain were firing electrical impulses, causing convulsions. Yet here there are no such impulses to be found. In epileptic seizures, brain waves form recognizable aberrant patterns on an EEG. In psychogenic seizures, patients' bodies shake, overtaken by tremors, but their monitored brain waves show no seizure activity. Their EEG patterns are consistent with an entirely alert and awake state.

Despite this measurable distinction on EEG, the diagnosis of psychogenic seizures is a notoriously difficult one to make and to treat. As the neurologist J. Chris Sackellares writes, detection of psychogenic seizures teaches 'the neurologist an important lesson in humility: even the best clinician can misdiagnose a pseudoseizure as an epileptic seizure or mistake an epileptic seizure for a psychogenic pseudoseizure'.

While Phyllis's body continued to shake, beating against the floor, I felt the full force of uncertainty as to whether her seizures were neurological or psychological in origin. I was flooded with a range of feelings, all of them uncomfortable. Tonight, as during each of the medical emergencies I had run to the previous two nights, I felt overcome by adrenaline's edgy, rattling buzz. During both of those scenarios, I fell back on the mantra of a life-support checklist: *Check the airway of the unresponsive woman. Ask the nurse to get her oxygen. Feel for a pulse – it's there, and strong. Get a set of vitals. Have the staff call rescue. This man is having a heart attack. Get him oxygen and aspirin. Have the nurse get a sublingual nitroglycerin out of the Pyxis. Get an ECG going. Call rescue. Call rescue. Call rescue.* When I first got to Phyllis, my mind began charting its way through seizure protocol, but a history of pseudoseizures complicated the picture and immediately shifted the course of action from clear to murky.

Ordinarily, with a patient still seizing as the four-minute mark came and went, I would administer a sedative – rectally, so the patient wouldn't spit it out or, worse, aspirate it or choke on it. I would call an ambulance to transfer her to the medical emergency room for status epilepticus. But Phyllis's history made it likely that she wasn't in status epilepticus, that she wasn't even having an epileptic seizure. In which case emergent transfer was not only unnecessary, it was contrathera-peutic. Given the fact that transfer to a medical hospital would likely mean administration of more and more sedating medications in an attempt to stop the seizure, it was also potentially dangerous.

As Phyllis's seizure continued, so did my unease. Her limbs and trunk thumped brutally against the floor, her head slamming over and over again into the thin hospital pillow. The staff members who stood around me shifted their gazes from Phyllis's convulsing body to me and back again.

'Five minutes,' the mental-health worker read from his watch. I sat quietly beside Phyllis, trying to will my stillness into her wild and unre-lenting movements. 'Six now,' he said. My heart was beating with such force that I felt it in my temples. I tried to reassure myself again and again, *Pseudoseizures. She has known pseudoseizures.* But what if this one wasn't? What if she were having an epileptic seizure? What if I were sitting – inert – beside her while she was going into status epilep-ticus and I did nothing to intervene?

'Okay,' I said. *Shit,* I thought. Close to seven minutes had passed. 'Somebody please call rescue, and let's give her the rectal diazepam. Who's holding arms and who's holding legs? The nurses are going to need some help to get it into her.' Immediately the room broke into motion. A mental-health worker ran out to make the phone call. Gloved hands held Phyllis to the floor by her wrists and ankles. A female nurse slid her hands beneath Phyllis's nightgown.

'In,' she said.

'Okay, great. You can let her go,' I said. The staff backed away from Phyllis. She continued to seize.

Another minute went by. Then three more. Then five. Phyllis was sweating badly now, her hair stuck in damp ribbons across her reddened face. The lack of effect from the medicine told me nothing; both nonepileptic seizures and status epilepticus can fail to respond to acute treatment. Finally, after several minutes more, I heard the clang of the unit doors opening to rescue's gurney and the deep voices of the EMTs. I began to stand, to go brief them on Phyllis, her history, the length of this seizure, the steps we had taken. As I did, Phyllis's shaking suddenly ceased. She opened her eyes and looked straight at me.

Rather than relief that her convulsions had finally stopped, I was surprised to feel mostly overcome by anger. I felt as though this woman had *fooled* me.

The EMTs rounded the corner and arrived at the Quiet Room's doorway. 'We're actually good,' I said to them. 'We're all set. You can cancel the rescue.'

'Cancel it?' the lead EMT asked.

'Yeah,' I said. 'Thanks for making it here so quickly. Sorry for the false alarm.' I stood, turned toward the door, and let out a deep breath, trying to defuse my anger.

The nurse in charge of the unit turned to me. 'Well, I guess she got her benzo, huh, Doc?'

I didn't answer. The implication in the nurse's comment was clear: Phyllis had pulled one over on us all. On me. I took another breath, then turned back around into the room. Phyllis sat herself up and was pushing her hair back out of her face.

'You all right?' I asked her.

'Yes,' she said quietly. 'Yes, I'm fine. After my spells I just need a little water and some rest. Or maybe someone could bring me some ginger ale?'

'Sure,' I said, trying to keep my voice calm so as not to show I was seething inside. 'Sure. We can get you some ginger ale.'

The diagnostic 'gold standard' – the most conclusive evidence – for psychogenic nonepileptic seizures is video EEG. In this test, patients are hospitalized, hooked up to electrodes that continuously monitor their brain activity, and simultaneously videotaped. To establish the diagnosis, the patient must seize while hospitalized and under these dual forms of observation. Then video-recorded seizure activity must be juxtaposed against the EEG reading of the same time period to show there is no epileptic activity on EEG. It's easy to imagine an aha moment that follows, where the detective/doctor swoops in at the end to reveal to the patient that he'll be fooled no more, the ruse is up. End of seizures, end of treatment, end of story.

As is true in most of medicine, the real narratives are not nearly so neat. First and foremost, establishing a diagnosis via video EEG is both difficult and costly. The seizure has to happen during the period in which the patient is hospitalized and under observation. Most patients' seizures are not predictable enough to ensure that the period of time required would be a reasonable one. Days of hospital treatment are staggeringly expensive, as is round-the-clock monitoring. For hundreds of thousands of Americans who suffer from psychogenic seizures (a recent estimate puts the range between 135,000 and 540,000), video EEG is not a realistic option. Even those patients who do receive a definitive diagnosis are not likely to capitulate and thus heal themselves. Patients may have little or no conscious awareness that their thoughts and feelings are driving their dramatic bodily responses. Although making patients aware that their seizures are psychological in origin is an essential component of treatment, it is rarely, in and of itself, curative.

The neuropsychologist Dalma Kalogjera-Sackellares describes the complexity associated with this shift in thinking by underscoring that for most patients with psychogenic nonepileptic seizures, their seizures have long been conceptualized by them, by their family members, even by their doctors as something they *have* rather than something they *do*. Once the diagnosis of psychogenic nonepileptic seizures is made, the role of psychotherapy is to help 'the patient realize, in a gradual and reasonable way, that spells are something a patient does in order to deal with something that disturbs him, [that] spells have a purpose in his life'. The goal of this reconceptualization is to shift the nonepileptic seizure from being a symptom of a disease to being a sign of distress, of difficulty coping. The ability to acknowledge and accept that shift, according to Kalogjera-Sackellares, is, 'in its own right, a strong positive prognostic factor. On the other hand, patients who continue to view their spells as having nothing to do with them psychologically have a poor prognosis'. If they will not acknowledge their seizures as psychologically based, they can't begin in earnest to discover what might be causing them.

These intersections of neurology and psychiatry are studied and treated by doctors in the specialized field of neuropsychiatry, a field that inhabits a narrow interspace at the confluence of psychiatry and neurology. Brown University neuropsychiatrist and behavioral neurologist W. Curt LaFrance Jr is a world-renowned expert in the treatment of neurologic symptoms that arise from psychiatric illness. He specializes in the diagnosis and treatment of conversion disorders, such as nonepileptic seizures and psychogenic movement disorders, in which psychic conflicts are converted into physical symptoms.

LaFrance underscores that the risks associated with misdiagnosis and overtreatment of psychogenic nonepileptic seizures – as when doctors misdiagnose a lengthy nonepileptic seizure as status epilepticus – can be grave. 'Complications of pseudostatus are iatrogenic', he writes. *Iatrogenesis,* from the Greek *iatro-,* 'physician', and *-genesis,* 'the origin'. This means that medical problems brought about by pseudo-status, or nonepileptic status, have nothing to do with the seizure itself but rather with the medical response to it. Iatrogenic complications, therefore, are caused by those of us whose Hippocratic edict is to first do no harm. According to LaFrance, these complications found in the medical literature include the effects and potential hazards of every single medical intervention employed. In order to stop a patient from seizing, doctors may insert catheters into major veins, which can bring about blood loss or infection. They may administer high-dose seda-tives, requiring patients to be intubated if their breathing slows too significantly. Rarely, through their interventions, doctors can cause respiratory arrest. 'Intubation is more common in pseudostatus rather than status epilepticus', LaFrance writes, because psychogenic nonepileptic seizures last longer and do not respond to antiepileptic drugs.

I met Dr LaFrance for lunch in a local bakery on an unseasonably warm November day to talk with him about my encounter with Phyllis and the mystifying nature of psychogenic nonepileptic seizures. Over sandwiches and gingerbread cake, Dr LaFrance explained that the dif-ficulty of distinguishing epileptic seizures from their nonepileptic counterparts is only part of the equation. The larger issue, he believes, has to do with the inherent discomfort doctors have with helplessness. In an emergency situation, how well can they sit with the fact that they cannot stop the patient from seizing? The answer is partially physician-dependent, of course, but it turns out for most of us the answer is . . . not too well.

'The psychiatrists are sometimes better at this than their neurology or emergency-medicine colleagues,' he began. 'You know, we neurolo-gists can inject you with medicine to bust a clot and reverse the effects of an oncoming stroke. A person can come into the ER with new-onset weakness or paralysis, and we restore full function with these powerful drugs. Emergency docs are used to performing that same kind of heroic intervention,' he said. I nodded. Of course this was true. My friends who are doctors in the ER often see my patients before I do. They empty a woman's stomach from her overdose and cleanse her liver from the toxins she ingested. They intubate her if she has taken enough pills or poison to stop breathing; they resuscitate her if her heart has stopped. They suture knife wounds, desperate and deep, that my patients have sliced into their arteries, then give their bodies back the pints of blood that they have lost. They find the lodged bullet from the self-inflicted gunshot that somehow missed its mark.

'So,' LaFrance continued, 'in the case of a nonepileptic seizure, it's incredibly hard for some doctors to sit with a patient and watch her suffering, when there is "nothing to be done".' *Don't just do something,* I think, *stand there.* 'We have this epilepsy algorithm, right? And on the side of seizures, we have a very specific set of steps to follow. We try this, and then we do that, and if that doesn't stop the seizure, we keep going down the line trying different interventions.' I nodded, thinking of the rectal sedatives I had administered to Phyllis when her convulsions weren't abating. 'On the other side of the algorithm, for nonepileptic seizures there is nothing to do. You wait it out. It's tough. The doctors watching a patient in status are between a rock and a hard place. They wonder, "If the seizure persists, could it cause damage?"' He paused. 'So what we see sometimes, as a result, are some patients with nonepileptic seizures who are intubated, paralyzed, put into medical comas because the doctor had to *do* something – she had to stop that seizure.'

LaFrance and others have written extensively about the costs of this iatrogenic harm, which, it turns out, is not at all uncommon. A 2003 paper in the *Journal of Neurology* reported that 27 percent of patients with unrelenting psychogenic nonepileptic seizures had been admitted to the intensive-care unit because doctors had mistakenly treated them for status epilepticus.

LaFrance summarized the issue by getting to the core of how medical students and doctors are taught to approach healing. 'I can stop your seizure,' he said, 'but can I be there – really *be* with you – as you are suffering?'

To describe this *being* with patients as they suffer, LaFrance employed a verb frequently used in a biblical context: 'to abide'. As in 'abide with' or 'abide by'. It is a powerful term that embodies diligence and, importantly, inaction. Its definitions, dating back to 1120, read like a recitation of devotion, a mantra of fidelity: 'to remain with, to hold to, remain true to. To endure, stand firm or sure. To wait till the end of, hear through. To await defiantly. To face. To encounter, withstand or sustain. To suffer, to bear, to undergo'. It is not, I suspect, a word that most people are inclined to associate with their modern-day medical care.

LaFrance believes that *abiding with* is central to the care and treatment of his complicated patients. 'They come to me,' he explained, 'and they say, "Doc, everyone told me you're the one who's going to cure me", and I say to them, "Well, they told you wrong, because I can't do that. But I can walk with you in this journey, and we can work together to understand what's going on that's causing you these problems that you've been having."'

I realized, listening to Dr LaFrance, that I had expected him to fill me in on cutting-edge treatments emerging in neuropsychiatry or to share with me some of his legendarily sharp diagnostic skills. I had thought he might direct me toward some new body of evidence from which his clinical success had come. Instead he had asked me to think about how well we as doctors can cope with the suffering of others and about how and why we distance ourselves from others' pain.

As we talked, I was struck by the tenuous position that Dr LaFrance occupies in a patient's treatment. Oftentimes he must deliver the news to patients that their seizures are in fact psychological, not neurological, in origin. I told him that I imagine people must, in response, feel angry, misunderstood, or ashamed.

'You have to help them understand,' LaFrance replied. And as he explained, I realized that by 'the' he meant both the population of patients suffering from nonepileptic seizures and the clinicians involved in their care.

First and foremost, LaFrance explained, clinicians must appreciate that patients with psychogenic nonepileptic seizures are not consciously trying to trick people. Their seizures are classified as a somatoform disorder, or a disease in which psychological symptoms manifest themselves physically.

On the other hand is a category of symptoms classified as malingering. 'Malingering is mendacity. It's lying,' he said bluntly. And he is right. In this category are prisoners who intentionally feign paralysis in order to be transferred out of prison and into a medical hospital or drug addicts who claim to be in extreme pain in multiple emergency rooms in order to acquire prescriptions for opiates. These are the patients who pretend not to know which hand holds the coin in Dr Charles Scott's coin-in-the-hand test. Malingerers make up fewer than 5 percent of the patients who seek treatment for somatoform symptoms. True somatoform disorders, in contrast, are not conscious and so do not fall into the category of deceit.

Nonetheless, just as I felt that Phyllis had fooled me, clinicians often feel duped by psychogenic nonepileptic seizures and other somatoform symptoms. This leads doctors and nurses to regard the somatoform illnesses as not real. Hence, for example, the historic classification of psychogenic nonepileptic seizures, catatonia, and other somatoform illnesses as hysteria. Hence the problematic and still-widespread nomenclature of *pseudo*seizures instead of psychogenic nonepileptic seizures. *Pseudo-,* from the Greek meaning 'false or falsely; to deceive or cheat'.

By the twentieth century, the prefix had come to designate whatever noun that followed it as pretended, counterfeit, spurious, a sham.

In *From Paralysis to Fatigue,* Edward Shorter reiterates the diagnostic point that unlike in malingering, there is nothing intentionally deceptive or false about somatoform disorders. 'From the patient's viewpoint', Shorter writes, 'psychosomatic problems qualify as genuine diseases. There is nothing imaginary or simulated about the patient's perception of his or her illness. Although the symptom may be psychogenic, the pain or the grinding fatigue is very real. The patient cannot abolish the symptoms by [simply] obeying the . . . injunction to [do so], for what he or she experiences is caused by the action of the unconscious mind, over which he or she by definition has no rational control'.

The fact remains, however, that patients who are told that the origins of their seizures are psychological rather than neurological may also wind up hearing this proclamation with the same implications of sham and deceit. LaFrance said he attempts to circumvent that outcome in the way he shares the diagnosis with patients. 'I focus on the fact that this is good news,' he explained. 'I tell them, "You don't have epilepsy." It's bad news to have abnormal brain-cell firing causing epilepsy. You don't want to have a tumor or something else that is anatomically wrong with your brain. So a diagnosis of psychogenic nonepileptic seizures should be reassuring. This is not some rare, never-before-seen collection of weird symptoms and spells. This is a clinical entity that is well understood and treatable. This is something that we can work on and fix.'

As Dr LaFrance spoke, I was reminded of the psychologist Stanley Standal, who argued that for therapy to work in any meaningful way the therapist must hold his patient in unconditional positive regard. Not unlike the parental or spousal ideal of unconditional love, a refusal to judge makes the therapeutic relationship a safe one in which very deep, often primitive conflicts may be revealed. Dr LaFrance offers just this kind of space by not judging his patients. The hope that Dr LaFrance and his patients share is that, through their work together, the patients' psychic conflicts – which have become so severe as to take shape in seizures or paralysis – can emerge to be dissected and made plain.

Therapists and doctors are human, of course. And thus this non-judgmental stance is neither effortless to employ nor consistently offered. Patients may unwittingly play into our own discomforts, our own insecurities.

As my lunch with Dr LaFrance drew to a close, I told him the story of Phyllis: the blue buzzer, her violent seizure, my confusion as to how best to proceed.

'What were you feeling in the moment?' he asked me.

I paused to consider the question, then answered. 'Fear,' I said.

'Fear of what?' he asked.

A torrent of responses ran through my mind: That I was missing something. That I should have been doing something differently. That Phyllis would decompensate as a result of my inaction and be in real, lasting danger. That the staff would see that I had mishandled an emergency and consider me an incompetent doctor. I told him these fears, or most of them.

'So her seizure became about you, huh?' LaFrance asked me gently, grinning. *I can stop your seizure, but can I really* be *with you as you are suffering?* Phyllis's seizure made me doubt my own capacity as a doctor, and my defensive reaction to that discomfort – and also that of the eye-rolling nurses – was to resent her, as if there were some malicious intent driving her to trick or mislead us. *Sham, falsehood, deceit.*

Dalma Kalogjera-Sackellares describes this perceived deception between doctor and patient in a mind-blowing but logical dynamic she calls the *double impostor scenario*. In this scenario, Kalogjera-Sackellares asserts, the patient responds to the news that his seizure or other somatoform disorder is 'not quite genuine' by feeling that he himself, as a patient, is therefore 'not a genuine patient'. Consequently the patient comes to feel 'like an impostor and his task, psychologically, at this point, will be to prove that he is not an impostor'. Proving that he is not an impostor may mean subconsciously causing his symptoms to escalate or developing new symptoms. It could mean calling into question the doctor's findings, intelligence, or credentials.

The double impostor scenario becomes even more wildly interesting as it begins to affect the patient's doctor, in whom, Kalogjera-Sackellares writes, 'a parallel psychological process is likely to occur'.

The doctor must face the 'sometimes very dramatic physical manifestations' of the patient's disorder, without the anchor of an identifiable physical illness. The doctor, Kalogjera-Sackellares writes, must first 'rule out a possible CNS (central nervous system) disorder. Even after this has been ruled out by an extensive evaluation, there may remain a lingering doubt that something was missed, or worse, that a CNS disorder can never really be ruled out in the future . . . with complete confidence. Thus, [the doctor faces] a situation which promises no real closure and which carries with it a threat of failure. Not being able to discover the underlying CNS pathology can make the neurologist feel like an impostor also, because the ability to perform that specific task is the unique contribution of his profession to medical science and is also one of the key aspects of his professional self-definition'. Hence the two impostors.

The patient, Kalogjera-Sackellares asserts, fears that the doctor will expose that he is not a true patient. The doctor fears he is not correctly assessing the patient's symptoms and that he will miss something neurological, which will expose that he is not a competent doctor. Kalogjera-Sackellares warns that this dynamic sets the doctor up not only for fear but also for shame. Shame is a more difficult feeling to manage psychologically than fear, so in defense, Kalogjera-Sackellares argues, clinicians transform their shame into anger. And they direct that anger toward their patients, as I did when Phyllis stopped seizing, opened her eyes, and asked me for ginger ale.

It seems obvious to say it, but what Kalogjera-Sackellares is getting at is this: It is hard to be empathetic and helpful to a patient if you see her as a threat to your credibility.

The risk of the double impostor scenario, or at the very least the risk that patients with somatoform disorders may be treated with mistrust and resentment, is a real and unfair one. And yet the historical treatment of these disorders – known collectively throughout previous centuries as hysteria – was far more grievous. Depending on the doctor and the era, hysteric patients were likely to be shown off, titillated, or terrorized.

The origins of the word 'hysteria' – from the Greek for 'womb' – squarely designate the illness as an exclusively female one. The seventeenth-century British physiologist William Harvey – who famously dissected the bodies of his own sister and father en route to discovering how blood was pumped through the body via the circulatory system – shared the widely held belief in the power of the uterus to wander about the body, wreaking both physical and psychological havoc. 'For the uterus is the most important organ', he wrote, 'and brings the whole body to sympathize with it. When the uterus either rises up or falls down, or is in any way put out of place or is seized with spasm – how dreadful, then, are the mental aberrations, the delirium, the melancholy, the paroxysms of frenzy, as if the affected person were under the dominion of spells, and all arising from unnatural states of the uterus'.

Despite not having a uterus, men were, and still are, afflicted with symptoms once deemed hysterical. The most widespread public example of this occurred during the First World War, when 'shell-shocked' men began to display symptoms of diagnoses that had always been relegated to women. Men were always as likely as women to have 'nervous breakdowns', but their symptoms – even if identical to those in their female counterparts – were more often deemed 'nervous' than 'hysterical'. Mark Micale, a medical historian and the author of the book *Hysterical Men,* explained in a *Smithsonian* magazine interview that there was a period of time in eighteenth-century Great Britain when it was almost fashionable to be a hysterical man.

'It was acceptable to acknowledge these symptoms in men and call them "nervous",' Micale confirmed. 'The label was applied, and self-applied, to men who were upper-middle or upper class, or aspired to be. They interpreted these symptoms not as a sign of weakness or unmanliness but as a sign that they had a refined, civilized, superior sensibility. . . . If you tire out easily, it's not because you're unmanly, it's because you have a particularly sophisticated nervous system that your working-class counterparts do not.'

Nonetheless, the majority of patients diagnosed with such hysterical disorders – psychogenic nonepileptic seizures included – have always been female. Hence the treatments for hysterical symptoms, developed almost entirely by male physicians, focused on the female reproductive organs and genitalia.

From the ancient era of Hippocrates to Galen and then continuing well into the twentieth century, physicians routinely employed a treatment for hysteria that is highly ironic in retrospect: Doctors would massage the genitals of their female patients until they responded with a 'hysterical paroxysm', after which point their symptoms would subside. The 'paroxysmal state' was, of course, an orgasm, and the written descriptions that persist recounting these events render it nearly impossible to believe that the majority of clinicians over the centuries did not recognize it as such, and yet they apparently did not. Galen, for example, in the second century A.D., described the resolution of a patient's symptoms after genital massage that resulted in contractions and the expulsion of fluid from the vaginal orifice. Seventeen centuries later, the American gynecologist William Goodell believed that vulval massage should be used to 'relieve pelvic congestion' in hysteric patients. Rachel Maines, in her always compelling and often hilarious book *The Technology of Orgasm,* deadpans of Goodell, 'His patients reported a desire to sleep after treatment.'

Maines describes how physicians, in an attempt to reduce the time spent on genital massage in their practices, led the quest to develop and market the vibrator. Medical practitioners remained utterly oblivious to the sexual nature of their treatments, a fact that Maines attributes to the 'androcentric' view of the times, in which women were thought to be sexually aroused and fulfilled only when penetrated.

This misconception gave rise not only to the blasé and clinical view of female genital massage but also to a spate of laughable fears that surrounded the invention of the speculum. As the nineteenth century drew to a close, 'any object or device that traveled the path of the totemic penis into the vagina was . . . suspected of having an orgasmically stimulating effect', Maines writes. 'The widespread adoption of the speculum as a medical instrument was far more controversial than that of the vibrator a few years later. Elaborate tales were related of women and girls lusting after medical examination and climaxing on the examining table the minute the speculum was introduced.'

Though speculum-induced climaxes are hard to imagine, Maines makes clear that climaxes were indeed happening through the other treatments. In 1653, Pieter van Foreest opined in his *Observationum et Curationum Medicinalium ac Chirurgicarum, Opera Omnia,* 'When these symptoms indicate, we think it necessary to ask a midwife to assist, so that she can massage the genitalia with one finger inside, using oil of lilies, musk root, crocus, or [something] similar. And in this way the afflicted woman can be aroused to the paroxysm.'

Delegation of the task to midwives was a means of saving physicians time, effort, and frustration deriving from the seemingly complex task of stimulating women's genitals. Maines writes, 'The job required skill and attention; Nathaniel Highmore noted in 1660 that it was difficult to learn vulvular massage. He said that the technique "is not unlike that game of boys in which they try to rub their stomachs with one hand and pat their heads with the other."'

Several less appealing treatments were devised to coax the wayward uterus back into place. Women with hysterical symptoms were made to sit above burners that wafted supposed womb-attracting fumes up into their nether regions. All manner of plants and oils were inserted into women's bodies to treat hysterical diagnoses ranging from insomnia and fainting to nervousness and convulsions.

It comes as no surprise, then, that massage-based treatments proved to be the more popular approach. As demand for massage grew, so did the amount of office time a physician could spend bringing his female clientele to their hysterical paroxysms. Rachel Maines writes that 'there is no evidence that male physicians enjoyed providing pelvic massage treatments. On the contrary, this male elite sought every opportunity to substitute other devices for their fingers, such as the attentions of a husband, the hands of a midwife, or the business end of some tireless and impersonal mechanism'.

That mechanism was the vibrator, conceived of and developed by a nineteenth-century British physician as a 'capital-labor substitution option', which 'reduced the time it took physicians to produce results from up to an hour to about ten minutes. . . . Mechanizing this task [of genital massage] significantly increased the number of patients a doctor could treat in a working day'. Samuel Spencer Wallian agreed in 1906, stating that massaging a patient by hand 'consumes a painstaking hour to accomplish much less profound results than are easily effected by the [vibrator] in a short five or ten minutes'.

Soon vibration treatments were not only available in the home but advertised widely in various upstanding women's publications. 'In the first two decades of [the twentieth] century', Maines writes, 'the vibrator began to be marketed as a home appliance through advertising in such periodicals as *Needlecraft, Home Needlework Journal, Modern Women, Hearst's, McClure's, Woman's Home Companion,* and *Modern Priscilla.* The device was marketed mainly to women as a health and relaxation aid, in ambiguous phrases such as "all the pleasures of youth . . . will throb within you". An especially versatile vibrator line was illustrated in the Sears, Roebuck and Company *Electrical Goods* catalog for 1918. Here an advertisement headed "Aids That Every Woman Appreciates" shows a vibrator attachment for a home motor that also drove attachments for churning, mixing, beating, grinding, buffing, and operating a fan.'

Though there is a decidedly comical element to treating somatoform disorders with vibrators and orgasms, far more sinister and less benign treatments were also employed. Had Phyllis's seizures occurred in the nineteenth century, she might as easily have been treated drastically, ineffectively, and possibly catastrophically with surgery. Though physicians largely agreed that the locus of female hysteria was the womb, the approaches as to how best to treat the trouble with the genitals diverged sharply. In *From Paralysis to Fatigue,* Edward Shorter writes that 'it was a short step from seeing genital lesions as the cause of mental disease to repairing them as a cure for it. And in one of the most audacious leaps in the history of nineteenth-century medicine, that is exactly the step that was taken. Gynecologists began operating on their patients to cure hysteria and insanity in an era that knew no antibiotic drugs against infection and that took only cursory precautions with surgical cleanliness'. Indeed, half of all surgical patients in the 1830s and 1840s died either during surgery or postoperatively, from surgical complications.

Yet swiftly and without substantial challenge, the field of psycho-gynecology was born. A procedural approach to treatment, which began with local 'remedies', such as carbolic-acid washes of the vulva, vagina, and cervix, evolved and gave way to major operations in which women's abdominal cavities were opened and their reproductive organs were surgically altered or removed. In the name of treating hysteria, hysterectomies were performed, uteruses were sewn to the abdominal wall, clitorises were cut out, and scores and scores of ovaries were removed from women of all ages. And these measures were heralded as great advancements in the field of medicine. In the late nineteenth century, Alfred Hegar, a professor of gynecology at the University of Freiburg, touted gynecology as 'the bridge between general medicine and neuropathology'. In this spirit, Hegar removed the ovaries of a twenty-seven-year-old who had complained of severe menstrual pain. She developed a postoperative infection and died shortly afterward from peritonitis. Nonetheless – and despite documented evidence of women's psychiatric illnesses persisting or worsening after surgery – physicians' enthusiasm for removing women's ovaries trundled on. It spread across Europe and across the Atlantic to America, where asylums hired staff gynecologists to perform pelvic surgery on their psychiatric inpatients.

Edward Shorter points out that male hysterics – of which there were many – were not routinely treated with castrations. Their physicians apparently – and no doubt accurately – presumed they would not like it: 'Archibald Church, a neurologist at Northwestern University . . . said in a discussion at a joint meeting of obstetricians and other specialists in 1904: "Men do not accept mutilating operations upon the genital tract with the equanimity which is presented by the gentler sex, who peaceably accept unsexing operations without much question as to their effect, provided they can be relieved of some trivial or temporary ailment."'

After I left Phyllis's floor, having written a note for the morning doctors and made sure she got her ginger ale, I headed back to my post in the psych ER. The overnight nurse, Ellen, was there, talking with José, a mental-health worker, about the latest change in the Red Sox pitching rotation.

'So what was the big emergency?' Ellen asked.

'Pseudoemergency,' I responded.

'Oh, you're kidding!' she groaned. Then she hit José lightly on the arm. 'Hey, remember that doozy of a pseudoseizure we had in here a couple of years ago? That woman we seriously thought was gonna die? It was wicked hot. Like July or something. Remember? At first we thought she was on drugs, then we thought it was the heat – '

'Oh, my God!' José interrupted. 'I *totally* remember. That woman was foaming at the mouth, and it did *not* stop, just kept going and going.'

'There were all these other patients around.' Ellen turned to me, filling me in on the story. 'And they started freaking out. Going, "What did you give her? What kind of place is this?" Like we had poisoned her or something.'

Then José jumped back in. 'And remember that guy . . . my God, it had to be four, five years ago, the one who kicked a hole in the door with his heel? *That* time I was sure it wasn't a pseudoseizure . . .'

They went on, swapping stories. Psychogenic nonepileptic seizures have long been viewed in this way – as a kind of spectacle – dating back at least as far as the nineteenth century and Jean-Martin Charcot.

Charcot, one of the most charismatic figures in medical history, fueled the nineteenth century's focus on hysteria. As the chief of neurology at the Salpêtrière Hospital in Paris, he became internationally known and revered as the master of diagnosis and treatment of hysteria. Letters sent from across the world needed only to be addressed to 'Charcot . . . Doctor in Europe', and they would reach him.

Charcot was uniquely situated to conduct research on women who were mentally ill. In 1880 he wrote, 'Among the five thousand female inhabitants of this great institution called the hospice of the Salpêtrière were a large number admitted for life as incurable, patients of every age with every kind of chronic disease, in particular disorders having the nervous system as their seat.' He made no bones about classifying his patients as objects for his scientific perusal. 'We found ourselves', he continued, '. . . in possession of a kind of living pathology museum whose holdings were virtually inexhaustible'.

In the midst of his 'museum' full of hysterics, Charcot developed an elaborate study of what he called 'attacks of hystero-epilepsy', a more sensational and arguably less authentic variation on today's psychogenic nonepileptic seizures. His patients would convulse, faint, flit in and out of consciousness, cry out with piercing wails, flail about their beds, exhibit pelvic thrusting, become immobile in the position of prayer or crucifixion, or strike Charcot's emblematic pose of hysteria: the *arc-de-cercle,* or *arc-en-ciel,* in which only their heels and the backs of their heads would be touching the ground.

Charcot's few critics and detractors cited 'hystero-epilepsy' as an illness that had been invented, not discovered, at the Salpêtrière. They accused Charcot of developing a culture of suggestion in which women were admitted with vague complaints and then continually exposed to other patients' behavior and symptoms. Eventually the women exhibited symptoms that conformed to Charcot's prized diagnosis and were rewarded with his interest and the encouragement of the staff. Ostensibly to silence his critics, Charcot began holding lectures and demonstrations to which the public was invited. He would let the people see this disorder, he said, and decide for themselves whether they believed in his ability to identify, induce, and treat hysteria.

Charcot's 'spectacles' became a notable destination for education, but mostly for entertainment. Axel Munthe, a psychiatrist and student of Charcot's who eventually became his critic, described the scene in detail, and not without derision: 'These stage performances of the Salpêtrière before the public of . . . Paris were nothing but an absurd farce, a hopeless muddle of truth and cheating. Many of [the patients] were mere frauds, knowing quite well what they were expected to do, delighted to perform their various tricks in public, cheating both doctors and audience with the amazing cunning of the *hystériques*. They were always eager to *"piquer une attaque"* of Charcot's classic *grande hystérie, arc-en-ciel* and all, or to exhibit his famous . . . stages of hypnotism, . . . all invented by the Master and hardly ever observed outside the Salpêtrière. Some of them smelt with delight a bottle of ammonia when told it was rose water, others would eat a piece of charcoal when presented to them as chocolate. Another would crawl on all fours on the floor, barking furiously when told she was a dog, flap her arms as if trying to fly when turned into a pigeon, lift her skirts with a shriek of terror when a glove was thrown at her feet with a suggestion [that it was] a snake.'

Despite Charcot's view of himself as an explorer of new psychiatric and neurological territory, his stance on the etiology of his patients' symptoms conformed to the prevailing theories of the day. Like his colleagues in Europe and beyond, he believed that the problematic locus of hysteria was the ovary. When a patient at the Salpêtrière who had been plagued by hysterical symptoms died, Charcot would largely ignore the brain in the autopsy, instead examining the ovarian tissue under a microscope for pathologic clues. His proposed remedies also targeted the ovaries. Charcot believed (and repeatedly demonstrated) that a hysterical attack could be made to cease (or sometimes begin) simply by the exertion of pressure on the ovaries. To that end, one of his interns developed a fit-preventing 'ovarian compressor belt' that supposedly applied constant pressure to these organs.

Ultimately, however, Charcot's sweeping power (if not his reputation) was limited to his lifetime. The Viennese psychoanalyst Wilhelm Stekel is quoted as saying, 'Twenty years after Charcot's death one could not find a single case of hysteria in any of the Paris hospitals.'

To learn more about somatoform disorders that might previously have been classified as hysterical, I shadowed Dr LaFrance one day in his neuropsychiatry and behavioral-neurology clinic. I watched him evaluate Gloria, a nineteen-year-old woman who had developed an incapacitating movement disorder over the past year. Before Gloria's appointment had even begun, I was aware of her symptoms. Sitting in the waiting area with her father, she was occasionally besieged by a violent jerk of one arm, accompanied by a forward thrust of her neck and a throaty, guttural honk. As she walked down the hall toward the exam room, the jerking and honking happened twice more. Passersby turned toward the noise and openly gaped at her.

In the exam room, with the door closed behind her, Gloria immediately started crying. Dr LaFrance had simply asked her to talk about what brought her to see him. Her body, so recently overtaken by dramatic spasms, sank into the more familiar convulsions of sobs as she described the gradual onset of her 'tics'. At first, about a year earlier, she had noticed her hand jerking occasionally, 'nothing that anyone would notice', she said. However, as weeks went by, the movements became more frequent and more pronounced.

'Suddenly my whole arm would jump across my body,' she explained through her tears, 'and then my neck started straining with it.' The movements weren't occasional anymore; they were happening many times in an hour, sometimes even every minute or so. They also weren't subtle anymore, and people began to turn to look at her.

'I used to go out with my friends,' Gloria said, 'but I stopped because I was so embarrassed.' The less she went out, the worse the movements became when she did leave the house. When the noise started in conjunction with the movement, Gloria and her family became distraught.

'Kids started pointing at me in the grocery store. People stared at me wherever I went. Sometimes I think I scared them. I'd be walking down a sidewalk or through a mall, and people would veer away from me. Or they'd put their arms around their kids and pull them quickly in the opposite direction, like I was contagious, or a crazy person or something.' Gloria had been working as a clerk at a rental-car company but left the job. 'They didn't fire me or anything, but they were worried about how customers would feel, whether it would turn people away. Once the noise started, I knew I didn't really have a choice. I couldn't stay.'

Dr LaFrance took a detailed history of Gloria's medical and psychosocial past. I was struck by the even and professional demeanor he maintained while conveying empathy. Gloria initially denied major stressors in her life but did admit that her parents' recent divorce weighed on her. She glanced frequently and guiltily at her father during the series of questions but acknowledged that she felt disloyal to one parent when spending time with another. She felt that her mother had become increasingly distant in the last couple of years.

Gloria's voice cracked as she spoke. 'I understand why she doesn't want to be with Dad, but I don't understand why she doesn't want to be with me.'

I felt sorry for Gloria. In that moment she seemed more like a child than a young woman. And as I was watching her, I realized that for the last many minutes – maybe even as long as half an hour – she had not once been besieged by any of her tics. She didn't seem to notice. Eventually she paused after a particularly emotional response and said, 'This actually feels good to talk about.'

Dr LaFrance nodded. Gloria suddenly looked startled. 'I haven't had a tic in a while, have I?'

'I wondered if you noticed that,' LaFrance replied warmly. Then he continued with the interview and examination. When I spoke with him afterward, I was longing to have observed some in-the-moment cure.

'I couldn't believe it,' I said. 'First she denied feeling stressed about anything. Then she started talking. Really *talking* about her parents' divorce and about how she felt rejected by her mother, and the movements and noises suddenly *stopped*.'

Dr LaFrance gently brought me back down to earth. 'It's great that she had that response,' he began, 'and especially great that she noticed it herself. But I wouldn't expect her movements to stop completely at this point.' In fact, LaFrance cautioned, if a patient appeared to have been cured after one visit, the core issues that gave rise to the movements might not have been reached, rendering it likely that the symptoms would return over time.

Gloria's movements were symptoms of a somatoform disorder, like nonepileptic seizures. The treatment would therefore be similar to the treatment of psychogenic nonepileptic seizures. First Dr LaFrance would help her begin to understand that her condition was psychogenic rather than neurologic. Once she accepted that, then they would work together to try to understand the precursors in her life, the circumstances and the precipitants or stressors that gave rise to Gloria's symptoms, as well as the factors that were perpetuating the abnormal movements. Identification of these contributing factors would shape Gloria's treatment, which might involve individual, group, or family therapy. It might also include combined pharmacologic treatment of depression, anxiety, or other psychiatric illnesses that could exacerbate Gloria's symptoms.

In other words, despite my hopes and initial excitement, Gloria's treatment would be neither as dramatic nor as neat as a sudden cure.

'But, hey,' LaFrance interjected, 'it's a good sign for her treatment that she acquired some insight as readily as she did.' He paused. 'A good sign.'

Gloria's illness offers a clear example of how unfair and misguided it is when psychiatric symptoms are misinterpreted as volitional. There is a common and erroneous belief that psychiatric illness is not real, that mental illness is 'all in your head' and can therefore be cured by force of will. Such a belief has no credibility; stacks of scientific and anecdotal evidence oppose it. And yet even for psychiatrists – who know well the capacity of the diseased mind to produce problematic behavior – it can be a challenge to remember that a patient's actions may not be a reflection of his or her will. When my catatonic patient Joseph did not respond to Henry's or my attempts to wake him, it was difficult not to feel as if he were being intentionally obstructive. Gloria's symptoms reminded me that these afflictions – which may well be a body's desperate cry for psychological healing – frequently bring added pain and suffering to the person experiencing them. Gloria would never have chosen to have an awkwardly flailing arm, a jutting neck, and an intermittent honking cry. Their existence brought her humiliation. Her symptoms cost her a job. They kept her in her house and away from her friends. They robbed her of joy.

One of the most puzzling manifestations of these kinds of somatoform illnesses occurs when, instead of manifesting in symptoms reflecting the private stress of an individual, they bloom and emerge in an entire group of affected people. Examples of this kind of outbreak, now deemed 'mass psychogenic illness', have occurred across cultures, continents, and centuries, from Charcot's Salpêtrière to modern America.

In 1952 the *New York Times* reported one such event, with the headline 165 GIRLS FAINT AT FOOTBALL GAME; MASS HYSTERIA GRIPS 'PEP

SQUAD'. The story reported that at the end of the first quarter of a high-school football game, the Natchez, Mississippi, Tigerettes prematurely began to march out onto the field to perform the halftime routine that they had prepared. An announcement was made over the loudspeaker clarifying that it was not yet halftime and calling the girls back to the bleachers, at which point the girls began to faint, presumably from mortification. In a description more reminiscent of the review of an action movie than a journalistic piece, the *Times* article reads, 'Football players dodged ambulances and autos that raced across the gridiron to take the girls to a hospital. . . . "It looked like the race track at Indianapolis",' Mr Thornton Smith, a spectator, is quoted as saying. '"They fainted like flies. Men swarmed right around the girls, picking them up and taking them to the foot of the stands."' Calls for doctors issued forth from the loudspeaker. Apart from describing the mayhem of the scene, the *Times* reports next to nothing about the girls, who they were, or how they began to faint. Instead the article takes note that they were wearing 'snappy, gold-trimmed black jackets and white skirts'. The girls were diagnosed at the local hospital with 'overheating and mass hysteria' – and meanwhile, 'Natchez won the game, 21 to 8'.

Many of the earliest recorded incidences of mass hysteria were the 'dancing plagues', or 'dancing manias'. From the ninth to the sixteenth centuries, reports emerged periodically across Europe of groups of citizens who began to dance and could not bring themselves to stop. Sometimes the dancers were isolated, as was the case of the Swiss monk who danced himself to death in his monastery's cloisters in 1442. More often they thronged in groups. And though some of the descriptions seem to describe a bacchanal in which drunken dancers claimed they could not stop the party, many are accounts of whirling horrors. Villagers danced until their feet were bloodied and sinew was exposed. They screamed to bystanders for help. They prayed for succor. They danced until they collapsed. Some danced until they died. Some jumped into rivers for relief, only to drown therein. Figures range widely as to how many people actually perished from dancing manias, but the written history of the Imlin'sche family of Strasbourg claimed that as many as four hundred people had died in a 1518 dancing plague there. Another chronicle from that same outbreak reported a period in which fifteen dancers died every day. The medical historian John Waller estimates that from the eleventh to the sixteenth centuries 'several thousand [people] had probably succumbed to a terrifying compulsion to dance'.

It is not known why or how these outbreaks began. There are certainly some reports of 'contagion', when tormented dancers would travel from one town to another and in each village new townspeople would find themselves afflicted. Yet there are broad gaps of both geography and time between epidemics. Direct contact – or even word of mouth or lore – does not sufficiently explain the symptoms' occurrences.

In Asia a fascinating psychiatric phenomenon called *koro* has emerged from time to time over the last century. Beginning in 1907 but occurring as recently as in 1987, episodes have been described in which groups of men became convinced that their genitalia were shrinking from a contagious illness. Thailand, India, China, and Singapore – all have recorded episodes in which groups of men, from a collection of co-workers to the entire male populations of certain villages, have been overtaken by the belief that their penises are shrinking, shriveling up, or being pulled into their bodies. The victims believe that once their penises disappear, they will die.

According to Robert E. Bartholomew in his book on mass psychogenic illness, entitled *Little Green Men, Meowing Nuns, and Head-Hunting Panics,* episodes of *koro* can last 'from a few days to several months and can affect thousands' of people. Bartholomew writes, 'Those affected often place clamps or strings onto the precious organ or have family members hold the penis in relays until appropriate treatment is obtained'. The exact nature of 'appropriate treatment' varies. In 1985, in the midst of what Bartholomew deems 'a major penis-shrinking scare', an eighteen-year-old Chinese agriculture student described his encounter with *koro* and the treatment he received: 'I woke up at midnight and felt sore and numb in my genitals. I felt . . . [my penis] was shrinking, disappearing. I yelled for help, my family and neighbors came and held my penis. They covered me with a fishnet and beat me with branches of a peach tree. . . . The peach tree branches are the best to drive out ghosts or devils. . . . They were also beating drums and setting off firecrackers. . . . They had to repeat the procedure until I was well again, until the ghost was killed by the beating'.

Parents may diagnose their sons with *koro* in the midst of epidemics, and their protective measures may in fact do real harm. During a three-month outbreak in Darjeeling, India, some parents were noted to have 'tied strong thread to their young sons' penises'. They anchored the thread by then tying it around their sons' waists. As a result some children developed penile ulcers. Of the Darjeeling outbreak, Bartholomew writes, 'The panic reached such levels that medical personnel toured the region, reassuring people by loudspeaker. . . . Doctors measured penises at intervals to allay fears by demonstrating there was no shrinkage'.

In Nigeria a rather different form of 'magical genital loss' has been recorded as recently as 1990, in which men walking in crowds believe that incidental contact with other men can cause their own genitals to vanish. A Nigerian psychiatrist reported that a police officer brought two men in to be evaluated. One claimed that in walking past the other man on the street, he 'felt his penis go' and went to the police, claiming that the man, whose robes had brushed him as they passed one another, had caused his penis to disappear. The 'victim' called upon the police officer to settle the matter. The psychiatrist describes examining the man in front of the officer and the accused. When the man's anatomy was pronounced normal, the 'victim' responded as if his penis had at that very moment been returned to him, though apparently with some concern as to whether it 'would function normally' after its recent disappearance.

The *Daily Times of Nigeria* reported that men began walking 'in the streets of Lagos holding onto their genitalia either openly or discreetly with their hands in their pockets' to defend against having their penises vanish or be stolen in these chance encounters.

Comical as the symptoms may seem, the results were sometimes tragic. When a man believed that his penis and scrotum had been stolen, he would shout, 'Thief! My genitals are gone!' – causing a swarm of sympathizers to rally to his defense. A paper in the *Transcultural Psychiatric Review* reports that crowds would 'immediately take steps to punish the "genital thief" by beating, clubbing, or even burning' him, believing that 'the rougher the treatment, the more likely it was that the "thief" would relent and "return the seized genital".'

Similarly violent and tragic consequences have accompanied other outbreaks of mass psychogenic illness. In seventeenth-century Loudun, France, Jeanne des Anges, the mother superior of a convent of Ursuline nuns, fell in love with a priest named Urbain Grandier. Initially the mother superior attempted to punish herself and eradicate her feelings through mortification – the religious process of exacting penance by means of self-injury. Though Jeanne flagellated herself and prayed throughout the day, Father Grandier came to her, unbidden, in lust-filled dreams at night. She was consumed by guilt and was eventually overcome by a trancelike state in which her body succumbed to bizarre movements and her speech issued forth in tongues. In the midst of this transformation, the mother superior claimed that she had become possessed and that Father Grandier was to blame.

In the days and months that followed, several other nuns in the Loudun convent began demonstrating symptoms attributable to demonic possession. The women fell into hysterical fits of all sorts, trembling and calling out in tongues, vomiting up worms and hair. One nun claimed to have spit up a portion of the heart of a child who had been sacrificed by witches. The nuns' displays, and the attempts to stop them via exorcism, drew a great deal of attention to the convent. Visitors and community members, in a manner that would seem to foretell Charcot's demonstrations of hysteria in the Salpêtrière, would come to watch the spectacle of possession. Robert Bartholomew writes that the nuns 'used the public exorcisms to draw attention to [Father Grandier's] immoral overtures and [to their own] pious sufferings'. With the evidence of his devilish influence compounding for all to see, Father Grandier was formally accused of witchcraft and was burned at the stake.

Other convents in other countries and centuries fell victim to similar episodes of mass psychogenic illness. Bartholomew postulates that the atmosphere in a convent was one in which the young female inhabitants were subjected to numerous constraints and regulations that they were powerless to protest. Accusations of witchcraft, therefore, 'were often a way to settle scores under the guise of religion and justice'. To the horror of observers and religious figures alike, afflicted nuns 'released frustrations by using foul, almost blasphemous language, by engaging in crude sexual behavior such as rubbing private parts or thrusting their hips to denote mock intercourse'. Bartholomew describes outbreaks in other convents: Sixteenth-century Spanish nuns convulsed and began to bleat like sheep; in a different region of France, nuns 'meowed together every day at a certain time for several hours'.

Strict or otherwise unpopular priests were often targeted, but fellow nuns were not immune from blame. In Germany in 1749, a young nun was accused of causing convulsions and trances among her sisters. She was charged with sorcery and 'beheaded in the market place to the cheers of an enthralled crowd'.

Crowds gathered, too, to observe Cree and Ojibwa teenagers in a remote Canadian community in the 1970s. The teens would fall into hysterical fits and run into the woods or hold their breath until they were given artificial respiration. The displays became a cause for the community to gather and to watch. Refreshments were served. Unsurprisingly, as long as the audiences persisted, so, too, did the symptoms. When the refreshments and gatherings were halted on the advice of psychiatrists, the fits suddenly halted as well.

As recently as 2012, girls in New York State were overcome by tics and other abnormal movements, prompting town residents (and eventually Erin Brockovich) to search for potential environmental causes for their new and terrifying neurological symptoms. The girls went on the *Today* show and were featured on the cover of the *New York Times Magazine*. Controversy swirled as to why – or whether – these popular, well-adjusted girls might be experiencing a mass psychogenic-movement disorder. As of this writing, no other definitive cause has been identified.

I n the same way that we understand individual somatoform disorders to be physical manifestations of psychic conflict, so group disorders are thought to arise in disempowered populations that lack other means of making their collective distress known. Hence nuns who gyrate and bark; hence young and overtired factory workers who begin, one by one, to convulse and collapse. Extrapolating further still, theories turn to political or sociological stress to explain cultural group afflictions: The medieval dancing manias occurred within the context of the Black Plague or during crop failures and resulting famines. Outbreaks of *koro* have tended to correspond with periods of economic fragility or political unrest. And yet, what of the subjugated millions who do not begin clamping their penises or dancing themselves to death? What of the war-torn countries that yield no groups of convulsing citizens? And how great was the degree of mass distress, really, of erroneously marching out after the first quarter to perform a halftime routine in snappy, gold-trimmed black jackets and white skirts? The theories feel as if they are trying too hard to fit. They do not snap into place with satisfying clicks.

When I told Dr LaFrance that I wasn't entirely convinced by these explanations of powerlessness, he shrugged. 'One deer in a group perceives a threat and its tail goes up. Another deer reacts. It bolts. And suddenly the whole group takes off like a shot.' He cautioned me, 'Don't forget we're also animals.'

O ne late-winter evening, it is barely dusk and I am driving my children home from swimming lessons. They are buckled into their car seats, wrapped in terry-cloth sweatshirts, and smelling of chlorine. A library audiobook plays for the hundredth time out of the car speakers. I realize with horror that I can recite this story, in which siblings travel through time and end up in a monastery in the Alps training Saint Bernards. I think, *If I have to listen to this story one more time . . .*

Outside the car window, strip malls and chain restaurants slide by in the gray-purple light of February. 'Why are swim lessons in Massachusetts?' my daughter asked once with a fatigued sigh, though the drive across the border takes us fifteen minutes tops. *Why indeed?* I think as we pass a Chili's restaurant and Walmart and iParty.

Then, just as the stoplight ahead flips to red and the brother and sister in the story magically turn into Saint Bernards to better save a fallen French soldier from an avalanche, my son points out his window, toward the sky, and says, 'Mama, what is *that?*'

My gaze follows his finger, and high above us, aloft, is a murmuration of starlings in flight. I cannot begin to guess their number. There are hundreds. Or thousands. They form a dark and undulating cloud, now condensing, now diving, now rising like a black swirl of smoke above the low winter sun. As they shift and morph, their individual selves are lost in the mesmerizing glory of the whole.

'Birds,' I say. 'It's birds,' my confused grammar reflecting the very question of the thing.

'Birds?' my children repeat with a gasp, incredulous.

'Look closely,' I tell them. 'The cloud is made up of birds. They're starlings, and they do this sometimes,' I say. 'They do this kind of dance.'

'Why?' my son asks, predictably.

"I don't know.' The light turns green, and as I start through the intersection, they protest immediately.

'Mama! Mama, stop! We can't see them if you do that!' So I pull over, into the driveway of a self-storage facility. I put the car in park. And while my children are otherwise captivated, I sneak my hand to the console and switch off the drone of the time-traveling sibling rescuers.

For a long moment, we watch quietly as the birds, in unison, glide and fall and rise. Then my daughter: 'Mama? Why does one of the birds turn?'

'What do you mean?'

'I mean, don't you think that one bird starts it? Don't you think that one bird decides they should go up instead of down or this way instead of that way, and it turns?' she asks me excitedly. 'And then the other birds follow?'

'Yes,' I say, 'I do think that's what happens.'

'Why does one turn, then?' she asks me. 'And why do the rest follow?' Yes, what small motion dictates where the group will go? What inclination strikes any single bird to lead?

'It's a good question,' I tell her. She is not satisfied with my answer.

'But *why*, Mama? I *really* want to know.' Her voice trembles. She is tired from swimming, from keeping her little body afloat, and she is hungry for dinner, and the inadequacy of my response has led her to the cusp of tears.

'I want to know, too, little bee,' I say.

'So do I,' my son pipes in softly. We sit still, in silence, watching the birds. Eventually, one by one, they land on a power line. They squeeze in beside each other. The children shriek in delight, as if landing birds are a miracle. The starlings have transformed, yet again, into some new shape. The line of them stretches down the road as far as we can see.

Into the Fire,
Into the Water

*And when they were come to the multitude, there
came to him a certain man, kneeling down to
him, and saying, Lord have mercy on my son: for
he is a lunatick and sore vexed: for ofttimes he
falleth into the fire, and oft into the water. And I
brought him to thy disciples, and they could not
cure him.*

– Matthew 17:14–16

It's been several years now since I was a resident, dreading blue
buzzers, a lone doctor in the psych hospital in the dead of night.
And the days of the consult service and Lauren's desperate ingestions
have begun to feel far away. Nonetheless, there have been countless
occasions since then, in the midst of my current practice, when I have
reminded myself of what I learned from Phyllis's seizure, or from
Anna's courage in trusting her ability to care for her son, or from
Joseph's utterly despondent body that could not even respond to pain.

The body mystifies. The mind more so. Witnessing their complex
intersections – and the unbidden ways in which the two can catastrophically fray – can unmoor us. As doctors, who must dwell daily at

the center of this unraveling, we can be tricked by action into feeling that our own human selves are less vulnerable. Yet action has the capacity to displace humanity, to disrupt connection, and, worse, to deceive. We reverse illness and cheat death often enough in the lives of our patients that we think we will surely be able to do so in our own. If we're moving, then we can't be caught. Yet our illusion of invulnerability is exactly that: an illusion. Like Colin's euphoric sense of love emanating from everything, invulnerability is a chimera that portends an eventual fall.

I can walk with you in this journey, Dr LaFrance tells his patients, whose bodies reveal the psychological pain beneath. He offers an alternative to action's false promises. I think often of how I left Joseph's side when he could not answer my questions, unnerved as I was by the silence. *I can sit with you in your pain,* I wish I could go back and tell him. *Or at least I am learning to.*

The poet Theodore Roethke endured episodes of severe depression throughout his life. His poem 'In a Dark Time' reads in part:

> *What's madness but nobility of soul*
> *At odds with circumstance? The day's on fire!*
> *I know the purity of pure despair,*
> *My shadow pinned against a sweating wall.*
> *That place among the rocks – is it a cave,*
> *Or winding path? The edge is what I have.*

As a psychiatrist, I hear the stories my patients tell me – noble souls that they are – and learn how their circumstances are at odds with their lives. They come to me bruised and upended, and when they do, the trajectories of their lives seem to them to be at best uncertain, at worst doomed. To fear that you might kill your own child, to scour your face with sandpaper, to swallow bedsprings – this is 'the purity of pure despair'.

If I am to abide with these patients, then I must accompany them to that place among the rocks, to the sweating wall. I must face with them the uncertainty of what lies beyond. I must stand at the edge with them and peer over into the fathomless depths. If I tell my patients, as I do, that this life can be a tolerable one, that they can face their fears and their traumas, their visions and voices, their misery, then I must look at what I am asking them to endure and I must look at it full in the face.

One recent Saturday morning, I sat down with a patient named Elizabeth who had been admitted hours before in the middle of the night. At home she had found herself lying in bed beside her husband imagining ways she could die that would look as if her death had been an accident rather than a suicide.

'I was so terrified by the thoughts,' she told me, 'that I stood up, changed out of my nightgown, and drove myself here.' She paused and then continued. 'Plenty of times recently, I've wondered why I'm still alive and whether it would be easier to die,' she explained, 'but I've never thought of actually killing myself before. I mean, I love my family . . . and that would be unforgivable after all we've been through. It would devastate them.'

'All you've been through?' I asked.

Tears slipped out of the corners of Elizabeth's eyes. Despite the tears, her voice remained steady and her expression was one of determined stoicism.

'Eight months ago,' she began, 'my son, Derek, was walking home from his high-school football game when he was hit and killed by a drunk driver. His sister had just started university, and she took it really badly. They were very close. We insisted she go back to campus. She'd worked so hard to get into her dream school and had been so happy there before . . .' Elizabeth trailed off. I waited for her to continue.

'I think we all hoped she would find solace in getting back to her routine, but she's really struggling with the death, and she says she feels so far from us. Then my husband lost his job – nothing he could have done about it, the company he'd been with for seventeen years was bought up and dismantled – but it was terrible timing. In this economy he's had no luck finding something else. And then there's my mom.' She laughed a self-conscious laugh through her tears. 'Not to totally open up the floodgates, but my mother has dementia, and I've taken care of her for the last two years, and it's gotten very hard lately. I don't know.' Elizabeth paused. 'My husband's of the mind-set, you know, "Everything happens for a reason", and "We've all got our crosses to bear", and "You can't move on if you dwell on things". But then I'll find him, for long stretches every day, staring at the computer, not typing or anything, just staring . . .' She took a deep breath and looked at me. 'I don't even know what I'm talking about. Isn't this pathetic?'

'It sounds like you're talking about loss,' I said softly.

Elizabeth's lips quivered, and her gaze turned to the crumpled tissue she was smoothing over and over again on the table between us. 'A year ago?' she began. 'A year ago I was dealing with my mom and I was joking to my friends about what a wreck I was going to be when my daughter moved away. I was happy for her, of course, but I knew I was going to miss her so much. You know what got me through it? My husband said to me one day, "Well, we had two years alone with her before Derek was born, and we loved those years. Now we'll have two years alone with Derek before he goes away to university." That was the thing I held on to when we drove away from her dorm. That I'd have two precious years to really *be* with my son, and then . . .' She began to weep. 'And then . . .'

I sat across from Elizabeth while she could not speak. Behind us I could hear the unit's washing machine begin to spin and a news program that some patients were watching on the television in the common area. I waited until she was ready to talk again. When she did, I listened.

Eventually she said, her voice breaking, 'Every minute when I wake up, I remember that Derek is dead. Every second of the day, I live with that knowledge – that loss – and I can't do *anything* about it. My son is dead, and my daughter is distraught, and all my life I've done everything I could to make them happy and strong, and there's not one thing I can do to change this for either of them. Not a thing.'

Elizabeth wept. She turned the tissue over to its other side and began to smooth it in the other direction. 'I miss my son,' she said. 'That emptiness never leaves me, not for a minute. And my husband can't talk about it, and my mother – who would have really *been* there for me – doesn't know up from down. And now I'm in a psych hospital because I keep thinking that I'd like to go to sleep and never – ' She choked a laugh and looked at me. 'Well, Dr Montross, I guess there's no direction to go but up now, is there?'

The French philosopher and Christian mystic Simone Weil wrote that to understand affliction one must accept our total human vulnerability. 'I may lose at any moment', she wrote, 'through the play of circumstance over which I have no control, anything whatsoever I possess, including those things which are so intimately mine that I consider them as being myself'.

Standing on the edge with my patients – abiding with them – means that I must harbor a true awareness that I, too, could lose my child through the play of circumstance over which I have no control. I could lose my home, my financial security, my safety. I could lose my mind. Any of us could.

A wonderful psychotherapist said to me, in the wake of my having learned of my mother's breast cancer, that we all live beneath a veil of invulnerability. For the most part, we act as if we and our loved ones will live forever. And then there are earthshaking moments in our lives – a diagnosis, an accident, some unforeseen catastrophe – when the veil is pulled back and we see with clarity that we are all in fact perched upon a precipice.

Mental illness pierces the veil, and those who suffer from it dwell with their fragility in plain view. My role as a psychiatrist is not to try to repair the veil but to strengthen my patients so that they can live, so that they can suffer less, so that they can hope.

Mary Weatherston is a psychologist who lives in Michigan. She is also a dear friend of mine. More than a decade ago, when I was trying to decide whether to go to medical school to become a psychiatrist, I called her to talk about her practice. I worried, I told her, about what it would be like to deal with my patients' misery day in and day out. In retrospect, I think I was asking her how to abide with the suffering of others.

Mary shares my love for northern Michigan and its lakes. Without thinking, she reached to that shared territory for a metaphor. 'The patients we work with have fallen through the ice in the middle of a frozen lake,' she began. 'My job – your job should you take this path – is to go out to them, to be with them on the thin ice, and to work with them to get them out of the frigid water.'

I listened as she continued. 'But you must know that if you go out to them on that thin ice, there's a real danger that you'll fall in, too. So if you go into this work, you've got to be anchored to the shore. You can reach out one hand to the person in the water,' she cautioned, 'but your other hand needs to have a firm grip on the people and things that connect you to the shore. If you don't, you lose your patients and you lose yourself.'

A short walk from the front door of our house is a path to the town beach. You turn the corner from a row of modest bungalows and Narragansett Bay suddenly appears at the end of a clearing, broad and commanding. The fateful names of its archipelago of islands seemingly chart settlers' initial promise and eventual desolation: Goat and then Starvegoat; Prudence, Patience, Hope, and then Despair. We moved to this sleepy neighborhood in part because Deborah could never see the logic to do otherwise. 'We live in the Ocean State,' she would say. 'Why would we not live near the ocean?' The minute we moved in a year ago, she vowed that she would see the ocean every day, and she has stuck fast to her promise. If she finds herself in the evening without having been to the water's edge, she will sneak down in the dark after the kids are in bed to breathe in the salt air. If it has been a daylong torrential downpour, she will slide behind the wheel of the car and drive the twenty seconds to the beach parking lot, where she will sit in the storm, windows cracked, and look out. I adore this about her. The insistence upon beauty and awe being a daily part of her life. The fixed principle of the thing.

What makes her devotion to the sea even more endearing is that she both loves and fears water. We were barely grown-ups when we met, twenty-four, full of passion and silliness and righteous indignation. I drove her up to my family's lake cottage in northern Michigan, where I discovered she could not swim, had never learned to do so. I taught her – floating, now face in the water and blowing bubbles, now gentle strokes and kicking all the while – and she loved it. But once she picked up her feet from the sandy bottom, she would giggle and tread water frantically, afraid to put them back down. Her abdominal muscles became rock hard that first summer. 'Panic belly', we laughed and called it, with the knowledge that our love, too, was new and deep and fearsome.

Fourteen years later, her love has grown, both for me and for the water. Our marriage is now a calming refuge, a profound entity we seem to have known intimately our whole lives. The ocean scares her still.

Recently Deborah took our borrowed kayak to paddle out into the bay. The water was calm, and she quickly ventured a fair distance from shore. I sat with the kids in the sand as they dug vast holes and collected hordes of vacant slipper shells. I watched Deborah's silhouette glide across the horizon, her winged paddles, the narrow body of the boat. From time to time, she'd turn and wave, smiling. Soon the water twenty feet in front of her began to ripple and splash. The bluefish were running, and we knew it. Fishers had come to plant their rods in the shoreline's firm sand, telling tales of bluefish so hungry they would beach themselves in an attempt to chase the glimmer of bait. In front of Deborah, the bluefish were after a group of sardinelike menhaden, churning the water into rough undulations that the fishers call a bluefish blitz. She looked back at me and pointed out to the choppy surface. I nodded. I had seen it, too. She paddled toward the shoal of fish, then floated, watching. The circle of churning water moved ten feet farther on. She paddled once or twice to follow them. Suddenly I looked up to see her paddling frenetically backward. The shoal had turned toward her. They were utterly harmless, but she wanted no part of being in the midst of their feeding. *Panic paddle.* I could not help but laugh.

We descend our neighborhood path not knowing how to interpret the signs the ocean offers us. One day a blanket of seaweed carpets the beach in a bright, luminescent green. The day before, tiny periwinkle snails were packed so densely on the ocean floor that it looked as if the sand were black. The day before that, the clear, calm shallows teemed with little hermit crabs that our children could clumsily catch, peer at, and let go. It baffles us, the ocean's rash showiness, its endless capacity for grand gestures and flux. It baffles all the more because it is paired with nature's silent and looming indifference. The still-feathered corpse of a seagull bobs on the incoming tide, head beneath the water and wings splayed across the surface. Or a wave tosses in a bleached vertebral column from what must have been a mighty fish. The wave recedes, the skeleton rolls on the shore, another wave washes over it.

One day as we are walking down the path, our daughter, newly in kindergarten, turns and asks me to carry her. She is exhausted, and she is sweet, and I love that she still has these moments when closeness is her only desire. I lift her to me with a mock groan, to which she says, 'Don't say I'm too heavy, Mama. I never want to be too heavy for you to carry me.'

'Someday you will be,' I say. 'When you are as big as me, you will be too heavy for me to lift! Maybe then you will lift *me*.' She laughs at this unimaginable thought, then quiets.

'How old will you be then, Mama?' she asks.

'When you are as big as I am?'

'When I am as old as you are now.' I do some quick math in my head.

'When you are thirty-eight years old, I'll be seventy,' I say.

She takes this in. She lays her head on my shoulder. 'Do you think you will live to be a hundred, Mama?' she asks me.

'I hope so,' I say, and squeeze her little body against me. It is the first time I am aware that she understands, if only a little, that I will some-day die.

'I hope you live to a hundred and three,' she says. She cannot see the tears welling up in my eyes. Through them the rolling bay ahead of us is foggy and shifting, even less well defined.

How do we do it? How do we bear the unbearable realities of our human lives? Someday I will die and leave Deborah, and our son, and our daughter. Or someday each of them will die and leave me. How do we reckon with this inconceivable a loss? With this cruel – and fundamental – truth? Perhaps we lift our feet off the ocean floor; we paddle frantically away from what we fear. Perhaps, for some of us, our very bodies revolt against what pains us. Our limbs convulse; our mus-cles suddenly weaken and fail.

I scan the beach. By what dumb luck do my lovely son and daughter have sound brains, good food, warm clothes, feather collections, wooden train tracks, two mothers who have loved them fiercely every second of their lives? Thus far we have been able to protect them from the deep and enduring traumas that scar the minds and selves of so many of the patients I see. How – *how* – can I make it always be so?

My children are off at a run, racing each other to some fast-chosen landmark. My daughter's arms flail alongside her; my son's little legs swing in determined, bowlegged arcs. She leads confidently, looking over her shoulder to giggle and gloat, until she snags her foot on a drift-wood branch and falls to the sand. She cannot decide whether she must cry. Her brother catches up, considers running on to the invisible finish line, then reconsiders and flops on top of her. They dissolve in laughter, roll so close to the water's edge that a wave nearly drenches them. They shriek, roll away from it, convulse with laughter, shriek some more. The sun is so bright on them it whites out the edges of their bodies. The sea retreats. My children roll out of the waves' reach. They roll onto their backs and pant, both looking up to the sky. Overhead, a lone gull flies above them, soaring, wings outstretched.

[ACKNOWLEDGMENTS]

The Brown University Department of Psychiatry and Human Behavior – and in particular my departmental chairperson, Dr Steve Rasmussen, and the directors of my residency training program, Drs Bob Boland and Jane Eisen – consistently helped me find ways to carve out time to devote to my writing. Dr Louis Marino guided me toward a professional schedule that made room for both writing and practicing psychiatry. I am exceptionally appreciative of such a supportive clinical home.

The MacColl Johnson Fellowship of the Rhode Island Foundation and the Eugene & Marilyn Glick Indiana Authors Award provided generous financial support to me as a writer. Bethlem Royal Hospital was kind to give me access to their voluminous archives.

Kris Dahl has been my advocate and adviser for almost a decade now. She is not only a wonderful agent but also my friend. I'm very grateful that she connected me with the good, smart people at The Penguin Press. Janie Fleming was enthusiastic about this book as my first imaginings of it began to form. Since that time the book has benefited by focused attention from Ann Godoff, Bruce Giffords, Scott Moyers, Maureen Sugden, and especially my editor, Lindsay Whalen. Lindsay asked all the right questions of the manuscript as I was writing it, and – as a good psychotherapist would – she didn't let me off the hook until she was sure I had found the core of what I wanted to convey.

Many of my colleagues enhanced my understanding of the illnesses and experiences I've written about in *Falling Into the Fire*. Ann Back

Price and Drs Colin Harrington, Martin Furman, Diana Lidofsky, Katharine Phillips, and Patricia Recupero are foremost among them, as is my friend and role model Dr Audrey Tyrka, who supervised my work with Anna and emboldened me to consider the case as one of anxiety rather than psychosis.

Conversations with Drs Carey Charles and Francis Pescosolido deepened my understanding of happiness and human vulnerability in immeasurably important ways. Dr Lawrence Price has been for me a mentor of the best sort: brilliant, encouraging, scrupulous, and irreverent. He read this manuscript through a meticulous and insightful lens. The fact that he is a member of the Michigan Wolverine faithful is icing on the cake.

I am fortunate to have good writers and good thinkers as friends, including Dr Jay Baruch, Peter Castaldi Sr, Dr Paul Christopher, Dr Kathryn Fleming-Ives, Kathleen Hughes, Lizzie Hutton, Kate Lorch, Alex Ralph, Leslie Smith, Maryll Toufanian, and Dr Alexander Westphal. Our conversations and their wisdom helped shape these pages. My poor friend Sheri Hook deserves particular mention, as she somehow always ends up reading the most outrageous and disturbing things I unearth in my research forays. I also appreciate Sarah Blaffer Hrdy's generous willingness to correspond with a stranger.

No book takes shape without essential pragmatic support. Elliot Fleming at the Brown Bookstore salvaged lost drafts and data that I had neglected to back up. Peter Shukat chased down elusive lyrics permissions so that I might have the very epigraph I wanted. And I am truly indebted to Maria Cervantes, whose kind attention to and care of my children is a gift beyond measure.

Dr Curt LaFrance Jr deserves special acknowledgment for sharing with me his thoughts about abiding with patients. My conversations with him transformed the trajectories both of this book and of my own psychiatric practice.

Being married to another writer is wonderful. Being married to another writer whose strengths compensate for your deficiencies is miraculous. From this book's first thoughts to its final line edits, it benefited from Deborah's unwavering and rigorous gaze. Indeed, it is not a stretch to say that inasmuch as the book succeeds in having a fluid and organic structure, it is a result of the many hours she spent arranging and rearranging my written lines, paragraphs, and pages to render my thoughts more lucid and my ideas more compelling and clear. Her steadfast devotion to me as a writer, as a parent, and as a partner is the single greatest treasure of my life.

Finally, I owe sincere thanks to my patients whose struggles inspired these narratives.

[BIBLIOGRAPHY]

Andrews, Jonathan, and Andrew Scull. *Customers and Patrons of the Mad-Trade: The Management of Lunacy in Eighteenth-Century London.* Berkeley: University of California Press, 2003.

Appignanesi, Lisa. *Mad, Bad and Sad: Women and the Mind Doctors.* New York: W. W. Norton, 2008.

Arnedo, Vanessa, Kimberly Parker-Menzer, and Orrin Devinsky. "Forced Spousal Intercourse After Seizures." *Epilepsy & Behavior* 16 (2009): 563–64.

Associated Press/*Huffington Post.* "Lashanda Armstrong, Distraught Mother, Drove Van Full of Children into Hudson River." *Huffington Post*, Apr. 14, 2011. www.huffingtonpost.com/2011/04/14/lashanda-armstrong-.distra_n_849141.html.

Bar-El, Yair, et al. "Jerusalem Syndrome." *British Journal of Psychiatry* 176 (2000): 86–90.

Barnes, Rachel. "The Bizarre Request for Amputation." *International Journal of Lower Extremity Wounds* 10 (2011): 186–89. PubMed, May 1, 2012.

Bartholomew, Robert E. *Little Green Men, Meowing Nuns and Head-Hunting Panics: A Study of Mass Psychogenic Illness and Social Delusion.* Jefferson, NC: McFarland, 2001.

Bayne, Tim, and Neil Levy. "Amputees by Choice: Body Integrity Identity Disorder and the Ethics of Amputation." *Journal of Applied Philosophy* 22, no. 1 (2005): 75–86.

Blom, Rianne M., Raoul C. Hennekam, and Damiaan Denys. "Body Integrity Identity Disorder." *PLoS ONE* 7, no. 4 (2012). www.plosone.org, May 1, 2012.

Bradshaw, Sarah. "Court, Cop Records Show Family Stress Grew Before Mom Killed Self, 3 Kids in Fatal Plunge." *Poughkeepsie Journal*, Apr. 16, 2011. www.poughkeepsiejournal.com/article/20110416/NEWS01/106270007.

Brozan, Nadine. "Lining Up for Hugs from a Guru of Touch." *New York Times*, July 8, 1998.

Camporesi, Piero. *The Incorruptible Flesh: Bodily Mutation and Mortification in Religion and Folklore.* Translated by Tania Croft-Murray. Cambridge, UK: Cambridge University Press, 1988.

Cappello, Mary. *Swallow: Foreign Bodies, Their Ingestion, Inspiration, and the Curious Doctor Who Extracted Them.* New York: New Press, 2011.

Carr, Marina. *By the Bog of Cats.* New York: Dramatists Play Service, 2002.

Christopher, Paul. "Safekeeping." *Brown Medicine*, Winter 2008, 38–44.

Ciotti, Paul. "Why Did He Cut Off That Man's Leg?" *Los Angeles Weekly*, Dec. 15, 1999.

Cojan, Y., et al. "Motor Inhibition in Hysterical Conversion Paralysis." *NeuroImage* 47, no. 3 (2009): 1026–37.

Cotterill, John A. "Body Dysmorphic Disorder." *Dermatologic Clinics* 14, no. 3 (1996): 457–63.

Dembosky, April. "Tour of Embraces Makes a Stop in Manhattan." *New York Times*, July 10, 2008.

Devinsky, Orrin, and George Lai. "Spirituality and Religion in Epilepsy." *Epilepsy & Behavior* 12 (2008): 636–43.

Devinsky, Orrin, Deanna Gazzola, and W. Curt LaFrance Jr. "Differentiating Between Nonepileptic and Epileptic Seizures." *Nature Reviews Neurology* 7, no. 4 (2011): 210–20.

Diagnostic and Statistical Manual of Mental Disorders: DSM-IV-TR. 4th ed. Washington, D.C.: American Psychiatric Association, 2000.

Dillard, Annie. *For the Time Being.* New York: Knopf, 1999.

Dominus, Susan. "What Happened to the Girls in Le Roy." *New York Times Magazine,* Mar. 11, 2012, 28–35, 46, 55.

Dotinga, Randy. "Out on a Limb." Salon.com, Aug. 29, 2012. www.salon.com/2000/08/29 /amputation.

Drury, M. O'C., and David Berman. *The Danger of Words: And Writings on Wittgenstein.* Bristol, UK: Thoemmes Press, 1996.

Elliott, Carl. "A New Way to Be Mad." *Atlantic Monthly,* Dec. 2000, 72–84.

Favazza, Armando R. *Bodies Under Siege: Self-Mutilation and Body Modification in Culture and Psychiatry.* 2nd ed. Baltimore: Johns Hopkins University Press, 1996.

———. "Treatment of Patients with Self-Injurious Behavior." *American Journal of Psychiatry* 147, no. 7 (1990): 954–55.

Favazza, Armando R., and Karen Conterio. "The Plight of Chronic Self-Mutilators." *Community Mental Health Journal* 24, no. 1 (1988): 22–30.

———. "Suicide Gestures and Self-Mutilation." *American Journal of Psychiatry* 146, no. 3 (1989): 408–9.

Favazza, Armando R., and Richard J. Rosenthal. "Diagnostic Issues in Self-Mutilation." *Hospital and Community Psychiatry* 44, no. 2 (1993): 134–40.

Feinberg, Todd E., et al. "The Neuroanatomy of Asomatognosia and Somatoparaphrenia." *Journal of Neurology, Neurosurgery & Psychiatry* 81 (2010): 276–81.

Fink, Max, and Michael Alan Taylor. *Catatonia: A Clinician's Guide to Diagnosis and Treatment.* Cambridge, UK: Cambridge University Press, 2003.

Fitzgerald, Jim. "NY Mom Who Killed 3 Kids in Hudson Is Laid to Rest." Oct. 1, 2012. abclocal.go.com/wpvi/story?section=news/national_world&id=8086002.

Ford, Charles V. *The Somatizing Disorders: Illness as a Way of Life.* New York: Elsevier Biomedical, 1983.

Freud, Sigmund, James Strachey, and Angela Richards. *On Psychopathology: Inhibitions, Symptoms and Anxiety, and Other Works.* Harmondsworth, Middlesex, UK: Penguin, 1979.

Fried, Ralph I. "The Stendhal Syndrome: Hyperkulturemia." *Ohio Medicine* 84, no. 7 (1988): 519–20.

Friedman, Susan H., and Phillip J. Resnick. "Mothers Thinking of Murder: Considerations for Prevention." *Psychiatric Times* 23, no. 10 (2006): 9.

Friedman, Susan H., et al. "Psychiatrists' Knowledge About Maternal Filicidal Thoughts." *Comprehensive Psychiatry* 49 (2008): 106–10.

Gabbard, Glen O. *Psychodynamic Psychiatry in Clinical Practice.* 4th ed. Washington, D.C.: American Psychiatric Publishing, 2005.

Gilman, Sander L. *Seeing the Insane.* New York: Wiley, 1982.

Giummarra, Melita J., John L. Bradshaw, Michael E. R. Nicholls, Leonie M. Hilti, and Peter Brugger. "Body Integrity Identity Disorder: Deranged Body Processing, Right Fronto-Parietal Dysfunction, and Phenomenological Experience of Body Incongruity." *Neuropsychology Review* 21 (2011): 320–33. PubMed, May 1, 2012.

Goode, Erica. "Suburb's Veneer Cracks: Mother Is Held in Deaths." *New York Times,* Mar. 2, 2011.

Gutheil, Thomas G. "A Confusion of Tongues: Competence, Insanity, Psychiatry, and the Law." *Psychiatric Services* 50 (1999): 767–73.

Guy, Melinda. "The Shock of the Old." *Frieze,* Nov. 20, 2009. www.frieze.com/issue/print _article/the_shock_of_the_old.

Haberman, Clyde. "Florence's Art Makes Some Go to Pieces." *New York Times,* May 15, 1989.

Hacking, Ian. *Mad Travelers: Reflections on the Reality of Transient Mental Illnesses.* Charlottesville: University Press of Virginia, 1998.

Haines, Janet, et al. "The Psychophysiology of Self-Mutilation." *Journal of Abnormal Psychology* 104, no. 3 (1995): 471–89.

Halim, Nadia. "Mad Tourists: The 'Vectors' and Meanings of City-Syndromes." In *Configuring Madness: Representation, Context and Meaning,* edited by Kimberley White, 93–108. Freeland, Oxfordshire, UK: Inter-Disciplinary, 2009.

Harlow, Harry F. "The Nature of Love." *American Psychologist* 13 (1958): 573–685.

Harlow, Harry F., and Margaret K. Harlow. "Psychopathology in Monkeys." In *Experimental Psychopathology: Recent Research and Theory,* edited by H. D. Kimmel, 203–29. New York: Academic Press, 1971.

Harlow, Harry F., and Stephen J. Suomi. "Social Recovery by Isolation-Reared Monkeys." *Proceedings of the National Academy of Sciences* 68, no. 7 (1971): 1534–38.

Harlow, Harry F., Robert O. Dodsworth, and Margaret K. Harlow. "Total Social Isolation in Monkeys." *Psychology* 54 (1965): 90–97.

Hatters-Friedman, Susan, and Phillip J. Resnick. "Child Murder by Mothers: Patterns and Prevention." *World Psychiatry* 6 (2007): 137–41.

———. "Neonaticide: Phenomenology and Considerations for Prevention." *International Journal of Law and Psychiatry* 32 (2009): 43–47.

———. "Parents Who Kill: Why They Do It." *Psychiatric Times,* May 2009, 3.

Hatters-Friedman, Susan, Sarah McCue Horwitz, and Phillip J. Resnick. "Child Murder by Mothers: A Critical Analysis of the Current State of Knowledge and a Research Agenda." *American Journal of Psychiatry* 162, no. 9 (2005): 1578–87.

Hatters-Friedman, Susan, Phillip Resnick, and Miriam Rosenthal. "Postpartum Psychosis: Strategies to Protect Infant and Mother from Harm." *Current Psychiatry* 8, no. 2 (2009): 40–45.

Hatters-Friedman, Susan, et al. "Child Murder Committed by Severely Mentally Ill Mothers: An Examination of Mothers Found Not Guilty by Reason of Insanity." *Journal of Forensic Science* 50, no. 6 (2005): 1466–71.

Hawton, Keith, et al. "Deliberate Self Harm: Systematic Review of Efficacy of Psychosocial and Pharmacological Treatments in Preventing Repetition." *British Medical Journal* 317 (1998): 441–47.

Hecker, Justus Friedrich Carl. *The Black Death and the Dancing Mania of the Middle Ages.* New York: Humboldt, 1889.

Hecker, Justus Friedrich Carl, and Benjamin Guy Babington. *The Epidemics of the Middle Ages.* Translated by B. G. Babington, et al. The Digital Collections: Cornell University Library.

Hrdy, Sarah Blaffer. *Mother Nature: Maternal Instincts and How They Shape the Human Species.* New York: Ballantine, 2000.

Ilechukwu, Sunny T. C. "Letter from S.T.C. Ilechukwu, M.D., Which Describes Interesting Koro-Like Syndromes in Nigeria." *Transcultural Psychiatric Research Review* 25 (1988): 310–13.

———. "Magical Penis Loss in Nigeria: Report of a Recent Epidemic of a Koro-Like Syndrome." *Transcultural Psychiatric Research Review* 29 (1992): 91–108.

Jamison, Kay R. *Night Falls Fast: Understanding Suicide.* New York: Knopf, 1999.

———. *An Unquiet Mind.* New York: Vintage, 1996.

Jay, Mike. *The Air Loom Gang: The Strange and True Story of James Tilly Matthews and His Visionary Madness.* New York: Four Walls Eight Windows, 2004.

Jean, F. Russell. "Dancing Mania." *Festschrift for Kenneth Fitzpatrick Russell: Proceedings of a Symposium Arranged by the Section of Medical History, A.M.A.* 1 (1977): 161–96.

Johnson, Eric Michael. "A Primatologist Discovers the Social Factors Responsible for Maternal Infanticide." Scientific American Blog Network, July 29, 2011. blogs.scientificamerican .com/guest-blog/2010/11/22/a-primatologist-discovers-the-social-factors-responsible -for-maternal-infanticide.

Kalogjera-Sackellares, Dalma. *Psychodynamics and Psychotherapy of Pseudoseizures.* Carmarthen, Wales: Crown House, 2004.

Karp, Joyce Gerdis, Laura Whitman, and Antonio Convit. "Ingestion of Sharp Foreign Objects." *American Journal of Psychiatry* 148, no. 2 (1991): 271–72.

Kenyon, Jane. *Otherwise: New and Selected Poems.* St. Paul, MN: Graywolf Press, 1996.

Khan, Abdus Samad, and Usman Ali. "Ingestion of Metallic Rods and Needles." *Journal of the College of Physicians and Surgeons Pakistan* 16, no. 4 (2006): 305–6.

Kleeman, Jenny. "Amma, the Hugging Saint." *Guardian,* Oct. 24, 2012. www.guardian.co.uk /world/2008/oct/24/religion-india/print.

Kreiser, B. Robert. "Religious Enthusiasm in Early Eighteenth-Century Paris: The Convulsionaries of Saint-Médard." *Catholic Historical Review* 61, no. 3 (1975): 353–85.

LaFrance W. Curt, Jr., and Orrin Devinsky. "The Treatment of Nonepileptic Seizures: Historical Perspectives and Future Directions." *Epilepsia* 45 (2004): 15–21.

LaFrance W. Curt, Jr., et al. "Cognitive Behavioral Therapy for Psychogenic Nonepileptic Seizures." *Epilepsy & Behavior* 14 (2009): 591–96.

McKee, Geoffrey R. *Why Mothers Kill: A Forensic Psychologist's Casebook.* Oxford, UK: Oxford University Press, 2006.

Maines, Rachel. *The Technology of Orgasm: "Hysteria," the Vibrator, and Women's Sexual Satisfaction.* Baltimore: Johns Hopkins University Press, 1998.

Marantz Henig, Robin. "At War with Their Bodies, They Seek to Sever Limbs." *New York Times,* Mar. 22, 2005.

Marx, Patricia. "The Stendhal Odyssey; Art Attack." *New York Times,* Aug. 20, 2000.

Masala, John. "Personality Disorder, Self-Mutilation, and Criminal Behavior." *Primary Care Companion Journal of Clinical Psychiatry* 11, no. 3 (2009): 123–25.

Masia, Shawn L., and Orrin Devinsky. "Epilepsy and Behavior: A Brief History." *Epilepsy & Behavior* 1 (2000): 27–36.

Menand, Louis. "Head Case: Can Psychiatry Be a Science?" *New Yorker,* Mar. 1, 2010.

Meyer, Cheryl L., Michelle Oberman, and Kelly White. *Mothers Who Kill Their Children: Understanding the Acts of Moms from Susan Smith to the "Prom Mom."* New York: New York University Press, 2001.

Morselli, Enrico. "Dysmorphophobia and Taphephobia: Two Hitherto Undescribed Forms of Insanity with Fixed Ideas." *History of Psychiatry* 12 (2001): 107–14.

Nicholson, Timothy Richard Joseph, Carmine Pariante, and Declan McLoughlin. "Stendhal Syndrome: A Case of Cultural Overload." *BMJ Case Reports* (2009). caserports.bmj.com /content/2009/bcr.06.2008.0317.abstract.

Nock, Matthew K. "New Insights into the Nature and Functions of Self-Injury." *Current Directions in Psychological Science* 18, no. 2 (2009): 78–83.

Oberman, Michelle, and Cheryl L. Meyer. *When Mothers Kill: Interviews from Prison.* New York: New York University Press, 2008.

Ogden, T. "On Projective Identification." *International Journal of Psychoanalysis* 60 (1979): 371–94.

Okeowo, Alexis. "A Once-Unthinkable Choice for Amputees." *New York Times,* May 14, 2012.

O'Sullivan, S. T., et al. "Deliberate Ingestion of Foreign Bodies by Institutionalised Psychiatric Hospital Patients and Prison Inmates." *Irish Journal of Medical Sciences* 103, no. 4 (1996): 294–96.

Patrone, D. "Disfigured Anatomies and Imperfect Analogies: Body Integrity Identity Disorder and the Supposed Right to Self-Demanded Amputation of Healthy Body Parts." *Journal of Medical Ethics* 35 (2009): 541–45. PubMed, May 1, 2012.

Phillips, Katharine A. *The Broken Mirror: Understanding and Treating Body Dysmorphic Disorder.* New York: Oxford University Press, 2005.

———. *Understanding Body Dysmorphic Disorder: An Essential Guide.* Oxford, UK: Oxford University Press, 2009.

Piers, Maria W. *Infanticide.* New York: W. W. Norton, 1978.

Porter, Roy. *Madness: A Brief History.* Oxford, UK: Oxford University Press, 2002.

Price, Lawrence H. "Letters – Looking at Ways to Treat Depression." *New York Times,* Jan. 11, 2010.

Pugnaghi, Matteo, et al. "'My Sister's Hand Is in My Bed': A Case of Somatoparaphrenia." Letter to the Editor, *Neurological Sciences,* Dec. 11, 2011.

Resnick, Phillip J. "Child Murder by Parents: A Psychiatric Review of Filicide." *American Journal of Psychiatry* 126, no. 3 (1969): 325–34.

———. "Murder of the Newborn: A Psychiatric Review of Neonaticide." *American Journal of Psychiatry* 126, no. 10 (1970): 1414–20.

Resnick, Phillip J., and Susan Hatters-Friedman. "Infanticide: Psychosocial and Legal Perspectives on Mothers Who Kill." *Psychiatric Services* 54, no. 8 (2003): 1172.

Roethke, Theodore. *The Collected Poems of Theodore Roethke.* Garden City, NY: Anchor Press, 1966.

Sacks, Oliver W. *The Man Who Mistook His Wife for a Hat and Other Clinical Tales.* New York: Perennial Library, 1985.

Saks, Elyn R. *The Center Cannot Hold: My Journey Through Madness.* New York: Hyperion, 2007.

Schachter, Steven C., W. Curt LaFrance Jr., and John R. Gates. *Gates and Rowan's Nonepileptic Seizures.* 3rd ed. Cambridge, UK: Cambridge University Press, 2010.

Schrom, T., and S. Amm. "Unusual Case of Oesophageal Foreign Body as Part of a Self-Harm Syndrome." *Laryngorhinootologie* 88, no. 4 (2009): 253–56.

Sedda, Anna. "Body Integrity Identity Disorder: From a Psychological to a Neurological Syndrome." *Neuropsychology Review* 21, no. 4 (2011): 334. PubMed, May 1, 2012.

Shapiro, David. *Neurotic Styles.* New York: Basic Books, 1965.

Shorter, Edward. *From Paralysis to Fatigue: A History of Psychosomatic Illness in the Modern Era.* New York: Free Press, 1992.

Solomon, Andrew. *The Noonday Demon: An Atlas of Depression.* New York: Scribner, 2001.

Sorene, E. D., C. Heras-Palou, and F. D. Burke. "Self-Amputation of a Healthy Hand: A Case of Body Integrity Identity Disorder." *Journal of Hand Surgery* (European Volume) 31, no. 6 (2006): 593–95. PubMed, May 1, 2012.

Spinelli, Margaret G. *Infanticide: Psychosocial and Legal Perspectives on Mothers Who Kill.* Washington, D.C.: American Psychiatric Publishing, 2003.

Starr, Mirabai. *Dark Night of the Soul.* New York: Riverhead, 2002.

Strong, Marilee. *A Bright Red Scream: Self-Mutilation and the Language of Pain.* New York: Viking, 1998.

Suyemoto, Karen L. "The Functions of Self-Mutilation." *Clinical Psychology Review* 18, no. 5 (1998): 531–54.

Taylor, Michael Alan, and Max Fink. "Catatonia in Psychiatric Classification: A Home of Its Own." *American Journal of Psychiatry* 160, no. 7 (2003): 1233–41.

Tucker, Abigail. "History of the Hysterical Man." *Smithsonian, Jan. 5, 2009.* www.smithsonianmag.com/science-nature/History-Of-The-Hysterical-Man.html.

United Press. "165 Girls Faint at Football Game; Mass Hysteria Grips 'Pep Squad.'" *New York Times,* Sept. 14, 1952.

Villalba, Rendueles, and Colin J. Harrington. "Repetitive Self-Injurious Behavior: A Neuropsychiatric Perspective and Review of Pharmacologic Treatments." *Seminars in Clinical Neuropsychiatry* 5, no. 1 (2000): 215–26.

Voon, et al. "The Involuntary Nature of Conversion Disorder." *Neurology* 74, no. 3 (2010): 223–28.

Waller, John. "Dancing Plagues and Mass Hysteria." *Psychologist* 22, no. 7 (2009): 644–47.

———. "A Forgotten Plague: Making Sense of Dancing Mania." *Lancet* 373 (2009): 624–25.

———. *A Time to Dance, a Time to Die: The Extraordinary Story of the Dancing Plague of 1518.* Thriplow, UK: Icon Books, 2008.

West, Sara G., Susan Hatters-Friedman, and Phillip J. Resnick. "Fathers Who Kill Their Children: An Analysis of the Literature." *Journal of Forensic Science* 54, no. 2 (2009): 463–68.

Zaroff, Charles M., et al. "Group Psychoeducation as Treatment for Psychological Nonepileptic Seizures." *Epilepsy & Behavior* 5 (2004): 587–92.

[INDEX]

abandonment, 50, 55
abiding:
    vs. active intervention, 177–79, 208
    as responsibility of doctors, 12, 179, 182,
        208–9, 211–12
abuse:
    child, 53–54
    in predisposition to self-injury, 47–48, 54
    sexual, 48
academia, madness seen as creative genius
    in, 109–13
accidental filicide, 142
acne, 68, 79, 81
addiction, to self-injury, 37
ADHD, 127
adrenaline, 6
aggression:
    and lack of bonding, 49
    of patients, 21–23, 38–43
alcohol, consumption of, 6–7, 21, 31, 35,
        36, 37, 100, 138, 142, 163, 171
altruistic filicide, 140–45, 158
American Journal of Psychiatry, 142, 154
Amma the Hugging Saint, 103,
        117–19, 133

amputation:
    BIID symptoms alleviated by, 87–88
    desire for, 12, 83–93
    ethical issues in, 85
    self-, 33, 49, 56–60, 85–86, 90
Amritaswarup, Swami, 118
Amsterdam, University of, 88
animal-rights movement, 48
Anna (obsessive-compulsive patient):
    diagnosis and treatment strategy for,
        157–61, 207
    potential for filicide by, 135–41,
        144–47, 150
anorexia, 69
antidepressants, 4, 29, 30, 67, 73, 76
antipsychiatry movement, 30
antipsychotics, 29, 108, 126, 130–31, 145
anxiety:
    in filicide, 150
    in intentional ingestion, 31
    in obsessive-compulsive disorder, 158–59
    postpartum, 150
    in tourists, 120, 122
apotemnophilia, 83
    see also body integrity identity disorder

arc-de-cercle (*arc-en-ciel*), 191–92
arm-drop test, 9–10
Armstrong, Lashanda, 155–56
art, psychotic reaction to, 121–23, 126, 132
Asia, *koro* in, 198–99
asomatognosia, 92–93
Ativan, 169
Atlantic, 83, 90
attachment theory, 53, 55
autism, 35
autonomy, 12, 89–90

bacchanals, 197
Bacchus (Caravaggio), 122
Baldwin, James, 111
Bar-El, Yair, 119–20
Bartholomew, Robert E., 198–99, 201
Baruch, Jay, 83
Baudricourt, Robert de, 130
Bayne, Tim, 87–89
BBC, 83
"bedlam," origin of term, 15
Bethlem Royal Hospital, xi, 1, 70
    brutal "therapeutic" treatment at,
        15–16
    "curable" vs. "incurable" classification in,
        14–15
    history of, 13–16
    as tourist attraction, 15
Bible, 34, 119, 121
biopsies, 31
bipolar disorder, 69, 103, 107, 108–9, 112
birds, group dynamics in, 203–5
birdwatching, 114–15
Black Plague, 202
Blaffer Hrdy, Sarah, 153–54
Blom, Rianne, 88
bloodletting, 16
Bodies Under Siege (Favazza), 34
body, intersection of mind and, 12,
        163–205, 207
body dysmorphic disorder (BDD),
        67–81
    BIID compared with, 84–85, 87
    causes of, 77–78, 83
    persistent, entrenched belief in, 80–81
    self-harmful consequences of, 72–75
    see also Eddie; Julie
body image:

erroneous self-perception about,
        12, 67–96
    identity and, 82, 85, 86, 93
body integrity identity disorder (BIID),
        83–93
    origins of, 91–93
    treatment for, 87–91, 93
    see also Corinne
Bondy, Philip, 85
bones, breaking of, 36
brain:
    effect of early trauma on, 47–48, 55
    mind and, 11, 181
    neurological function of, 8–9, 11–12, 78,
        92–93, 192
brain injury, 8, 12
breasts, self-amputation of, 35
Breathalyzer, 5, 98
Bright Red Scream, A (Strong), 53
British Journal of Psychiatry, 119
British Medical Journal, 123
Brockovich, Erin, 202
Brodie, Benjamin, 84
Broken Mirror, The (Phillips), 74
Brown, John Ronald, 85
Brown University, 40, 48, 53, 104, 176
Brunelleschi's dome, 123
Buddhism, 17
burial, alive, 70
burning, self-injury through, 12, 35, 36,
        75, 139
buzzer system, for emergencies, 166–69, 182

Calder, Alexander, 127
California, University of, at San Diego, 92
Canada, 201–2
cancer:
    of author's mother, 211
    treatment of, 129–30
Caplan, Art, 90
Cappello, Mary, 42
Caravaggio, 122, 126, 132
castration, 189
    female, 34
    self-, 33–34
catatonia, 11, 180, 196
    see also Joseph
Cello Concerto in A Minor
        (Schumann), 111

cellulitis, 166
Center Cannot Hold, The (Saks), 169
central nervous system (CNS), 183
Charcot, Jean-Martin, 190–93, 196, 201
childbirth, 151–52
child murder, *see* filicide
"Child Murder by Parents: A Psychiatric
    Review of Filicide" (Resnick), 142
children:
    abuse and neglect of, 53, 142, 144, 155
    of author, 6, 12–13, 61, 65, 82, 93–95,
        114, 130, 133, 147–53, 164, 203–5,
        213–16
    killing of, *see* filicide
    loss in death of, 209–11
    maternal harm to, 12, 135–61
China, 198–99
Christopher, Paul, 104
Church, Archibald, 189
Church of the Holy Sepulcher, 120
cigarettes, in self-mutilation, 35
city syndromes, 119–23
clinical intuition, 106
clitoris, 189
cognitive behavioral therapy (CBT), 80
cognitive function, 8
coin-in-the-hand test, 8–9, 180
Colin (spiritual euphoria patient), 97–109,
    116, 117, 119, 123–24, 131–32, 208
comas, 12, 178
command hallucinations, 33–35, 56,
    59, 164
    obsessive thoughts vs., 146–47
Complete Obsession, 83–84, 86
Comprehensive Psychiatry, 140
contagiousness, 198, 199–200
control, through dissociation, 52
conversion disorders, 176
Corinne (BIID subject), 84, 85,
    86, 93
cortisol, 150–51, 153
"Crazy" (Gnarls Barkley), 97
Cree tribe, 201–2
Crowder, J. E., 34
Cruise, Tom, 30
culture shock, 122
cutting, self-injury through, 12, 36, 49–53,
    75, 139
cysts, 32

Dadd, Richard, 15
Daily Times of Nigeria, 200
dancing plagues, dancing manias,
    197–98, 202
"dangerous wellness," 107
Dante Alighieri, 110
Darjeeling, India, 199
darshan, 118
Darshan: The Embrace, 117–18
Dawn (nurse), 139, 145, 159
death penalty, 155
Deborah (author's partner), 81–82
    author's relationship with, 6, 8, 61, 65,
        93–96, 130–31, 147–48, 151–52,
        212–16
    in parenting, 12–13, 65, 151–52
defense mechanism, humor as, 42–43,
    45–47
deformation, fear of, *see* dysmorphophobia
delirium, 166
delusions:
    in BIID, 97–133
    in filicide, 143
    paranoid, 15, 109, 115, 122, 123,
        124–25, 136, 143
    somatoparaphrenic, 91–92
    urge toward goodness in, 116–17, 128
    see also religious and spiritual delusions
dementia, 112, 210–11
demonic possession, 200–201
dentistry, 71, 74, 79, 86
depression, 1, 91, 106, 111, 113,
    195, 208
    in catatonia, 3–11, 16
    in ingestion, 31, 42–43
    medications for, 4, 29, 30
    misdiagnosis of, 30
    of mothers, 140
    postpartum, 30, 112
    suicide and, 39
    symptoms of, 4
Derek (Elizabeth's son), 209–11
dermabrasion, 68
dermatology, 68, 75
des Agnes, Jeanne, 200–201
"desiccation," 68
developmental disability, self-mutilation
    and, 35–36
devil, 15, 140, 143

Diagnostic and Statistical Manual of Mental Disorders (DSM), 84, 109
diazepam, 173–74
Dillard, Annie, 117, 132
disability, symptom exaggeration in applicants for, 8
disassociation, 122
disconnection, 32–33
disgust responses, 89–90
disintegration, 122
dissociation, in self-injury, 50–54, 55
divine experiences, 12
doctors:
    anger and resentment felt by, 37–38, 42–45, 174–75, 182–84
    consulting, 9–10
    coping mechanisms for, 42–43, 46–47, 100–101, 106, 179
    decision making by, 164–75
    ethical responsibilities of, 14, 25, 56–60, 85, 87–93, 119, 125–27
    frustation of, 26, 40–42, 44–45, 55
    as held accountable for failure, 78–79
    as imposters, 182–84
    inaction as counterintuitive for, 170–71, 177–79
    insurance company pressure on, 14
    lack of empathy in, 100–101
    primary-care, 6
    risks for, 27, 98–99
    vulnerability of, 6, 39–42, 136, 170–75, 180–84, 208, 211
    see also medicine; psychiatry
double imposter scenario, 182–84
draftees, symptom exaggeration by, 8
Drexler, Melissa "Prom Mom," 142–43
drugs:
    illicit use of, 21, 31, 35, 36, 37, 55, 103, 117, 138, 165
    overdose on, 7, 157, 168
    see also specific prescription and street drugs
Drury, M. O'C., 130
dysmorphophobia, 69–70
"Dysmorphophobia and Taphephobia" (Morselli), 70

ears, in BDD, 72
eating disorders, 37

ecstasy, psychosis vs., 12
Eddie (BDD patient), 67–71, 73, 75–81, 84
    trajectory of treatment for, 76–77, 79–81
ego-dystonic visions, 158
elective amputation, ethics of, 85, 87–93
electroencephalogram (EEG), 172, 175
Eliot, George, 107
Elizabeth (despondent patient), 209–11
Ellen (nurse), 190
Elliott, Carl, 83, 90
emergency room:
    author's experience with, 19–23, 97–99, 163–69, 190, 207
    patient evaluation for, 3–6, 20–23, 99, 101–2, 125, 137–38, 163–65
    treatment protocol for, 172–73
endoscopies, 24–25, 31, 58–59
enucleation, 33–34
epileptic seizures, 143, 170–71, 173–74, 177–79
euphoria:
    malignant potential of, 106–9, 131–32
    spiritual state of, 12, 101–7, 109
    see also Colin
Euripides, 135
evaluation, author's procedure for, 5, 7–8, 20–23
executions, 52
exorcism, 201
exposure therapy, 158–59
eyes, self-removal of, 33–34

face, in BDD, 71, 72
fainting, mass, 196–97
Favazza, Armando, 33–37
fear:
    author's experiences of, 93–96, 131, 149–52, 182, 215
    of doing harm, 135–40, 159
    heightened senses in, 6
    plans vs., 158
    in schizophrenia, 116
female genital self-mutilation, 34
fetters, in hospitalization, 16
filicide, 140–44, 208
    classification in, 141–43
    motivation for, 160–61
    in nature, 153–54

risk matrix for, 156–57
stress and, 150–54, 155
finger foods, 20–21, 28
fingers, in BDD, 73
Florence syndrome, 121–23
"foreign body," 32, 52
Foscolo, Ugo, 123
Fourth Amendment rights, 124–25
Fra Angelico, 122
Frankel, David, 53
Freiburg, University of, 189
Freud, Sigmund, 45
Friedrichs, Dr., 25
From Paralysis to Fatigue: A History of Psychosomatic Illness in the Modern Era (Shorter), 84, 181, 188
Frost, Robert, 19–20, 64
frostbite, 86, 88
Furth, Gregg, 84, 85

Gabbard, Glen, 52
gag reflex, 10, 16
Galen, 185–86
gangrene, 85
gastroenterology, 19–20, 25
gender dysphoria (gender identity disorder; transsexualism), 85
gender reassignment, 87
genetics, in mental illness, 78
genital massage, 185–88
genius, madness and, 110–13
Georgia, 105
Germany, 201
Gloria (movement disorder patient), 193–96
Gnarls Barkley, 97
God, in religious delusions, 34–35, 117, 131
Goodell, William, 186
Grandier, Urbain, 200–201
Great Britain, 78–79, 154–55
hysterical men in, 185
grief, dissociation in, 52–53
Guardian, 118
gynecology, 188–89

Haines, Janet, 50–51
hair, in BDD, 75
hair pulling, 36
Halim, Nadia, 121–22

hallucinations, 33, 35, 56, 59, 146–47, 166
hallucinogens, 103, 124
hand, self-amputation of, 56–60
Handel, George Frideric, 110, 111
Harlow, Margaret and Harry, 48–49
Harrington, Colin, 48
Harvey, William, 184
head banging, 36, 49, 170, 173
health insurance companies:
    clinical decisions influenced by, 14
    economics of, 30, 62, 74, 89, 99, 175
    shortcomings of, 56, 62–64
Hegar, Alfred, 189
helplessness, 202–3, 210–11
Hemingway, Ernest, 110
Henry (nurse), 5–10, 196
Highmore, Nathaniel, 187
Hinduism, 118
Hippocrates, 177, 185
homelessness, 127–28
homicide, 21
    of father, 15
homosexuality, as motivation for self-amputation, 35
hope, in BDD, 76–81
Hôpital Sainte-Anne, 121
hospitalization:
    admission to, 14, 37, 164–75
    involuntary, 12, 104–6, 163
    role of, 27
Hudson River, 155–56
hugging, Amma's use of, 118
humor, as coping mechanism, 42–43, 86–87, 100–101, 106
hurricane, as metaphor for life trauma, 93–96
hygiene, 4, 121, 124
hyperstates, 106
hypnotism, 192
hysterectomies, 189
hysteria, 184–89, 190–92
    mass, 196–203
Hysterical Men (Micale), 185
"hysterical paroxysm," 185
hystero-epilepsy, 191

iatrogenic harm, 177
"imagined ugliness," 69
Imlin'sche family, 198

"In a Dark Time" (Roethke), 208
India, 118–19, 198, 199
infanticide, 141–43
    laws pertaining to, 154–55
Infanticide Act (British; 1922), 155
infection, 21
inferiority, 78
infidelity, projection in, 45–46
intentional ingestion, 19–33, 42–43, 75, 207
    items swallowed in, 23–24, 25, 27–29,
        31–32, 42–43, 208
    self-injury by, 12, 21–29
    see also Lauren
Internet, 117
interpersonal conflict, 50
intubation, 177, 178
"Iron Rations: Fakirs Swallow Swords, but
    Amateurs Take Cake Lunching on
    Hardware," 42
isolation:
    body image in, 69, 71
    desire for, 11, 16
    early, 48–49
    in filicide, 155
    social, 194–95
Israel, 119–21

Jamison, Kay Redfield, 112
Jane 5 ward, 44
Japanese tourists, 121
Jehovah's Witnesses, 90
Jerusalem syndrome, 119–21
Jesus Christ:
    Colin and, 97–98, 101
    delusions involving, 34, 56, 59, 120
Jim and Wendy (author's neighbors), 95
Joan of Arc, 130
Johnson, Eric Michael, 150, 153–54
José (mental health worker), 190
Joseph (catatonic patient), 3–11, 12, 16–17,
    196, 207, 208
Journal of Abnormal Psychology, 50
Journal of Applied Philosophy, 88
Journal of Clinical Psychiatry, 34
Journal of Hand Surgery, 86
Journal of Neurological Sciences, 92
Journal of Neurology, 178
Julie (BDD patient), 74–75, 86
Justice Department, U.S., 141

Kalogjera-Sackellares, Dalma, 176, 182–83
Kay (grandmother's friend), 114
Kleeman, Jenny, 118
Klein, Melanie, 45
kleptomania, 37
koro, 198–99, 202

labor, 74
LaFrance, W. Curt, Jr., 176–83, 193–96,
    203, 208
Lauren (intentional ingestion patient),
    19–33, 207
    causes for disorder of, 50–51, 54–55, 56
    as chronically returning patient, 19, 29,
        31, 43–44, 54, 60–62
    compared with amputation patient,
        58–59
    failure of health care system for, 62–64
    family background of, 55
    hostility of, 21–23, 38–44, 46–47, 60
    projective identification as response to,
        46–47, 50
    superficial/moderate self-mutilation in,
        36–37, 59
    treatment strategy for, 31–33, 37–38, 51,
        54–55, 56, 59–64
learning disability, self-mutilation and,
    35–36
Lee, Nathaniel, xi
Levy, Neil, 87–89
Lidofsky, Diana, 53
lightbulbs, 19, 21–23
Literary Digest, 42–43
Little Green Men, Meowing Nuns,
    and Head-Hunting Panics
    (Bartholomew), 198
London Eye, 149
loss, death and, 209–11, 215
Loudun, France, 200
Lowell, Robert, 107, 110
"lunatics," 13

Macbeth (Shakespeare), 1
McGeoch, Paul D., 92–93
McKee, Geoffrey R., 156–57
Mad Pride, 110
"Mad Tourists" (Halim), 121–22
Maestripieri, Dario, 152–53
Magherini, Graziella, 122–23

"magical genital loss," 199–200
magnetoencephalography, 92
Maines, Rachel, 186–88
major self-mutilation, 33–35, 59
malingering, 8–9, 180–81
managed care, *see* health insurance companies
mania, 127–28, 130
  depression and, 106–7
manslaughter, vs. murder, 155
marijuana, 21, 103
Martha (tourist), 122
Mary, Virgin, 34
mass psychogenic illness:
  causes of, 202–3
  examples of, 196–202
"Maternal Filicide Risk Matrix," 156–57
Matthew, Book of, 33, 67, 207
Mayo Clinic, 72
Medea (Euripides), 135, 142
media, images of perfection in, 78
Medical and Behavioral Treatment Plan,
    26–28
medication:
  effective, 30, 125–26
  ineffectiveness of, 29–30, 88, 145
  for mental illness, 16, 23, 29, 103–4,
    119, 130–32
  misuse of, 127–28
  patient volition and, 12, 104, 105,
    108, 163
  reliable use as important in, 31, 67, 79,
    107, 116
  in seizure threshold, 171
  side effects of, 31
  see also specific drugs
medicine:
  author's evolving perception of, 1–2
  "cover your ass" (CYA) approach in, 165
  ethical issues in, 14, 25, 56–60, 85,
    87–93, 104–6, 119, 125–27, 131–32
  financial issues in, 14, 16, 29
  hierarchies of decision making in,
    164–75
  intersection of psychiatry and, 163–205
  judgment calls in, 128–30
  omission vs. commission in, 58–59
  potential treatment hazards in, 177
  shortcomings of, 17, 46–47, 77
  see also doctors; *specific disciplines*

meditation, 17
medulla, 10
Melancholy, 15
memories, personal, 13
memory loss, 8
men, and hysteria, 184–85, 189
mental illness:
  dangers of undertreatment of, 107–8
  drug use in, 7
  ethical issues in, 56–60, 131–32
  historical treatment and mistreatment
    of, 13–17, 188–89, 190–93, 197–98,
    200–201
  importance of correct diagnosis in, 12,
    146–47, 157–58, 166, 176–77, 182
  interdisciplinary conference on, 109–13
  myth of romantic madness in, 15,
    110–13, 132
  onset of, 115–16
  perceptual acuity in, 39–41, 136
  physical illness vs., 93, 129–30
  social circumstances vs., 29–30
  subjects as "spectacles" in, 15, 190–93,
    201–2
  see also specific disorders
Messiah (Handel), 111
Mexico, 85
Micale, Mark, 185
Michigan, author's fondness for, 65, 114,
    147, 212, 213
midwives, 186–87
migraines, 11
mind:
  as domain of psychiatry, 11–12, 17
  intersection of body and, 12,
    163–205, 207
  mysteries of, 12
minimal engagement, 4
mirrors, obsession with, 68–70, 80
misdiagnosis:
  dangers of, 12
  of depression, 30
Missouri, University of, 33
mockingbirds, 114–15
Molière, 163
Monica (manic patient), 127–28
monkeys:
  bonding research on, 48–49, 55
  cortisol and stress in, 152–54

Monro, Thomas, 16
Montross, Christine:
  contemplation of hard questions by, 1–3,
    16, 17, 90–91, 93, 112–14, 117, 119,
    126–33, 147–53, 203, 207–16
  doubts and unease of, 1–3, 16, 17,
    38–42, 44–47, 61–65, 77, 90–91,
    108–9, 110, 116, 131, 160–61, 165,
    168, 170–75, 180, 182, 212, 215
  evolving perceptions of, 1–2, 12–13,
    207–16
  grandmother of, 114–15
  hurricane experience of, 93–96
  mission of, 2–3, 39–40, 106
  motherhood of, 6, 12–13, 61, 65, 82,
    93–95, 114, 130, 133, 147–53, 164,
    203–5, 213–16
  parents of, 148, 211
  partner of, see Deborah
  presentation on theme of madness by,
    109–13
  psychiatry as career choice of, 2–3, 19,
    167–68, 208, 212
  residency of, 3, 19, 39, 67, 72, 99,
    163, 207
  as risk-averse, 164–65
mood disorders, 30
mood stabilizers, 29
Morselli, Enrico, 69–70
mortification, 200
Mother Nature (Blaffer Hrdy), 153–54
mothers:
  fears of, 149–53
  harming of children by, 135–61
  murders by, 141–44
movement disorders, 176, 193–96, 202
Mrs. Dalloway (Woolf), 111
Munch, Edvard, 110
Munthe, Axel, 192
murder:
  manslaughter vs., 155
  of one's own children, see filicide;
    infanticide
mutilators, 51
mystics, 12

nail biting, 36
Nancy (paranoid schizophrenic patient),
  124–26

Natchez, Miss., 197
natural selection, 150, 153
nausea, induced, 16
neglect:
  child, 53–54
  in predisposition for self-injury, 47–48
neonaticide, 141–43
nerves, 11
"nervous breakdowns," 185
Nervure, 121
neurological examination, 5–7
  symptom validity tests in, 8–10
neurology:
  BIID origins in, 91–92
  intersection of psychiatry and, 11–12,
    172, 175–84
neuropsychiatry, 176–84, 193
Neuropsychology Review, 92
New York, State University of, Buffalo, 117
New York State, 202
New York Times, 30, 118, 122, 196
New York Times Magazine, 202
New Zealand, 155
Nigeria, 199–200
nipples, in BDD, 73
nonhuman primate research, 48–49
nonmutilators, 51
nonsuicidal self-injury, 35
Northwestern University, 189
noses, in BDD, 72, 74–75, 86
nuns, 200–202
nurses:
  briefing role of, 3, 169
  functions of, 20, 169–70, 174
  resentment felt by, 37–38, 46, 174,
    182, 190

object relations theory, 45
Observationum et Curationum
    Medicinalium ac Chirurgicarum, Opera
    Omnia (van Foreest), 186
obsession:
  in BDD, 67–81
  in BIID, 90
  command hallucinations vs., 146–47
  of harming child, 135–40, 152, 158
obsessive-compulsive disorder, 36, 147,
  158–60
  see also Anna

ocean, as metaphor for life, 212–14
O'Connor v. Donaldson, 105
Ojibwa tribe, 201–2
"ominous extravagance," 106
One Flew Over the Cuckoo's Nest,
    105, 107
opiates, 7, 165, 180
    natural occurrence of, 50–51
orgasm, as treatment for hysteria, 185–88
Osiris, 15
ovarian compressor belt, 192
ovaries, 189, 192
Oxford English Dictionary, The, 69, 83

pain:
    assessing of, 9
    in BDD, 73–75
    as deterrent to self-injury, 33
    distancing from, 179
    as evaluative tool, 5–6, 8, 10
    lack of sense of, 35, 50–51
    as penance, 34, 200
    physical vs. psychic, 21–23, 47, 75, 86,
        202, 208
    physiological response to, 6
    in psychogenic disorders, 181
paralysis, 9
paranoia, 15, 109, 115, 122, 123, 124–26,
    143, 163
paraphilias, 83
parent-infant bonding:
    in attachment theory, 53
    research on, 48–50
parenting:
    author's experience of, 6, 12–13, 61, 65,
        82, 93–95, 114, 130, 133, 147–53,
        164, 203–5, 213–16
    psychiatry compared with, 13
    research on, 48–49
parietal lobe, 92–93
Paris, 190
Paris syndrome, 121
paternalism, 104
patients:
    abiding with, 12, 136
    antagonistic stance of, 21–23, 38–43
    autonomy issues and, 12, 89–90, 104–6,
        119, 125–27, 163
    briefing routine for, 3–4
    as chronically returning, 4, 14, 23–24,
        99, 157, 164
    classification of, 14
    doctors duped by, 6, 136, 170–75,
        180–84
    "gravely disabled," 105
    as imposters, 182–84
    nonjudgmental relationship to, 181–82
    palliative measures vs. cures for, 26
    premature discharging of, 14, 23
    resentment engendered by, 37–38, 42–45
    self-perception of, 102, 103
    self-reporting by, 50
    sense of loss in, 209–11
    short-stay, 13–14, 99
    threats of violence by, 78–79, 116,
        135–40
    vulnerability of, 2–3
    see also specific individuals
Patty (self-mutilation patient), 34–35
pediatricians, 7, 142
pedophilia, 136
penises:
    self-amputation of, 35
    shrinking and disappearing of, 12,
        198–200, 202
pep squad, mass psychogenesis in,
    196–97, 203
pharmaceutical companies, 30
phenothiazine, 130
Phillips, Katharine, 72, 73–75, 77–78, 81
Phyllis (seizure patient), 169–75, 177, 178,
    180, 182, 184, 188, 190, 207
Pierre, Jean, 155–56
Plath, Sylvia, 110, 113
polyps, 31
Ponte Vecchio, 123
possession, demonic, 200–201
postpartum psychosis, 30, 112, 157
postpartum stress, 150–51, 155
post-traumatic stress disorder (PTSD),
    169–70
poverty, 31
preaching, 121
pregnancy, stress during, 150
Price, Lawrence, 30–31
prodromal phase, 109
projection, 45–47
projective identification, 45–47, 50

prostitution, 55
Prozac, 79
pseudoseizures (psychogenic nonepileptic
    seizures), 171–80, 182, 185, 188, 195
  history of, 190–93
Psychiatric Times, 140
psychiatry:
  author's hard questions about, 1–3, 16,
      17, 90–91, 93, 112–14, 119, 126–33,
      147–48, 207–16
  difficulty of determining a diagnosis in,
      108–9, 126, 128, 132, 137, 146–47,
      157–58, 163–64, 166, 170–75,
      182–84
  doctor's nonjudgmental stance in, 181–82
  domain of, 11–12
  emergency procedures in, 166–69
  historic evolution of, 13–17
  intersection of medicine and, 163–205
  lack of certainty in, 168
  as medical discipline, 11
  mission of, 106
  myths and misperceptions about, 30–31,
      105, 107
  perceived as pseudoscience, 30
  responsibilities of, 3–4, 208, 211
  risks to practitioners of, 98–99
  shortcomings of, 106
  surgery vs., 26
Psychiatry: An Industry of Death, 30
psychogenic movement disorders, 176
psychogenic nonepileptic seizures
      (pseudoseizures), 15, 171–80, 182,
      185, 188
  history of, 190–93
psychogynecology, 189
psychology, 11
psychopharmacology, 30
"Psychophysiology of Self-Mutilation"
      (Haines), 50
psychosis:
  delirium vs., 165–66
  euphoria and, 106–8
  in harming of children, 140–41, 144–47
  obsession vs., 146–47, 158
  in self-mutilation, 33–35, 59
  see also schizophrenia
psychotherapy, 16
  for BDD, 73, 80

in BIID, 88
  for depression, 30
  for pseudoseizures, 176
  psychotic filicide, 142–43, 147

quadriplegics, 12
Quiet Room, 169–70, 174

racism, 143
Raving Madness, 15
rectal insertions, 35
reflexes, 8
Reid, Russell, 88
rejection, 50
religious and spiritual delusions, 56, 59,
      97–121, 126, 128, 130–33
  faith vs., 119
  in harming of children, 140, 143–44
  mass psychogenesis in, 200–201
  in self-mutilation, 33–35
  see also Colin
"Repetitive Self-Injurious Behavior: A
      Neuropsychiatric Perspective and
      Review of Pharmacologic Treatments"
      (Villalba and Harrington), 47–48
repetitive self-mutilation syndrome, 37
reproductive system, in hysteria,
      184–85, 189
research, ethics of, 48–50
Resnick, Phillip, 141–44, 147, 159–60
respiratory rate, 7
restraints, in hospitalization, 16
rhinoplasty, 72
Rhode Island:
  author's home in, 212–13
  hurricane in, 93–96
  involuntary hospitalization in, 104
Riggi, Theresa, 142
risk, author's avoidance of, 164–65
Roethke, Theodore, 208

Sackellares, J. Chris, 172
Sacks, Oliver, 106
saints, 12, 130–31
Saks, Elyn, 169
Salpêtrière Hospital, 190–92, 196, 201
Santa Croce, Church of, 123
Santa Maria Nuova Hospital, 122
Satan, 140, 143

scabs, reopening of, 36
schizophrenia, 69, 91, 103, 111, 116–17,
    168, 169
  and BIID, 108–9, 115–16
  catatonia in, 11
Schumann, Robert, 111, 113
Scientific American, 150, 153
Scientology, 30
Scott, Charles, 8–9, 180
scrotums, 200
Sears, Roebuck and Company
    catalog, 188
seclusion, 169–70
security guards, 20–22, 28–29, 39,
    40–41, 98
sedation, sedatives, 5, 7, 29, 30, 173–74,
    177, 178
Sedda, Anna, 92
seizures, 7, 12, 143, 170–76, 178, 180, 182,
    188, 207
  see also Phyllis
self-amputation, 33, 49, 56–60, 85–86, 90
self-fulfilling prophecy, projective
    identification as, 45–47
self-help, morbid forms of, 36
self-image, self-harm and, 67–96
self-injury, 19–65, 165, 200, 208
  anger and resentment at, 37
  disconnection in, 32–33, 50–54, 55
  ethical issues in, 56–60
  feedback loop in, 36–37, 59
  through ingestion, see intentional
    ingestion
  involuntary hospitalization and, 104
  normal aversion to, 32–33
  physiology of, 51
  root causes of, 47–50
  through self-mutilation, 33–37
  sense of calm and relief through, 33, 36,
    47, 49–51, 75
  sequence of events in, 50–51
  three types of, 33
  as unintentional consequence of BDD,
    72–75
self-mutilation, 33–37
self-soothing, 53
Selma (BDD patient), 79
sensory loss, 9
separation, self-injury prompted by, 50

September 11, 2001, terrorist attacks of,
    52, 145
serotonin, 78
serotonin reuptake inhibitors (SRIs), 76,
    79–80
sex:
  body identity and, 85
  irregular actions and desires in, 83,
    139, 201
  as motivation for self-injury, 34, 35, 200
  perceived relationship of hysteria to,
    184–89
Sexton, Anne, 110, 112
sexual abuse, 48, 53–54
Shakespeare, William, 1, 19
shame, in doctor-patient relations,
    183–84
Shelley, Percy Bysshe, 110
"shell-shocked," men, 184–85
Shorter, Edward, 84, 181, 188
short-stay patients, 13–15
sigmoidoscopy, 35
Simon, Robert I., 116
sinfulness, as motivation for
    self-mutilation, 34
Singapore, 198
skin, in BDD, 67–70
Slater mental hospital, 44
Smith, Robert, 85, 88
Smith, Susan, 143
Smith, Thornton, 197
Smithsonian, 185
snapshots, residents' game with,
    99–101, 106
somatoform disorders, 180–84, 193–96
  throughout history, 184–88
  misinterpretation of, 196
somatoparaphrenia, 91–93
sparrow, 115
speaking in tongues, 200–201
spinal cord, 11
spouse-revenge filicide, 142, 144
Standal, Stanley, 181
starlings, group behavior of, 203–5
status epilepticus, 170–71, 173–74,
    177, 179
Stendhal syndrome, 123
stereotypic self-mutilation, 33, 35–36
sternal rub, 5–6, 8

"Stopping by Woods on a Snowy Evening" (Frost), 19–20, 64
Strasbourg, 198
stress:
    cortisol and, 150–51
    ingestion as response to, 23–24, 31, 33, 46–47
    of isolation, 48–49
    in mothers who harm children, 152–54, 155–57
    self-mutilation as response to, 36–37, 51
    social, 31, 154
    in somatoform disorders, 194–95, 202–3
stroke, 7, 11–12
Strong, Marilee, 53
stupor, 11
subcision, 81
submersion, as therapy, 16
suicide:
    attempted, 21, 115–16
    in BIID, 99, 106
    as consequence of BDD, 73, 77, 79
    drug overdose in, 7
    and filicide, 138, 139, 144, 155–56
    genius and, 112
    hospital precautions for, 27
    passive, 73
    self-injury vs., 33
    tendencies toward, 1, 29, 86, 88, 107, 122, 164, 209
    threats of, 39, 166
superficial/moderate self-mutilation, 33, 36
superglue, 72
Supreme Court, U.S., 105
surgery:
    ability to cure by, 26
    for amputation, 56–60
    author's dream about, 41–42
    cosmetic, 68, 72, 73–74, 75–77
    dental, 71
    as effective in BIID, 83–84, 86–93
    historical dangers of, 188–89
    for ingested objects, 19, 23–27
    self-, 72
Swallow: Foreign Bodies, Their Ingestions,
        Inspiration, and the Curious Doctor
        Who Extracted Them (Cappello), 42
symptom exaggeration, 8–9
symptoms:
    tests for neurological validity of, 8–10
    see also specific symptoms
Szasz, Thomas, 30

Taking of the Christ (Caravaggio), 132
Technology of Orgasm, The (Maines), 186
teeth, in BDD, 71, 74, 79, 86
testicles, self-amputation of, 35
Thailand, 198
"Thorazine shuffle," 105
thyroid, 21
tics, 193–94, 202
Today, 202
Tourette's disorder, 36
tourists, psychotic episodes of, 119–24
tranquilizers, 171
Transcultural Psychiatric Review, 200
transformation, 126–27
transgendered people, 35
trauma:
    dissociation and, 52–53
    neurological effects of, 47–48
    retelling of story as reexperiencing of, 145–46
Troilus and Cressida (Shakespeare), 19
tumors, 32

Uffizi gallery, 122
unemployment, 31, 209–11
unresponsiveness, 5–11, 17
    obstructionist, 11
unwanted child filicide, 142–43, 144
Ursuline nuns, 200–201
USA Today, 118
uterus, in hysteria, 184, 187, 189

Vancouver ferry, 149
van der Kolk, Bessel, 47–48
van Foreest, Pieter, 186
van Gogh, Vincent, 110, 113
veterinary medicine, 7
vibrators, 186–88
vigilance, maternal, 151, 153

Vijay (medical student), 102–3
Villalba, Rendueles, 48
vital signs, 5, 7
voices, hearing of, 15, 56, 83, 109, 115,
    116, 138–39, 144–46, 166
vulval massage, *see* genital massage

Waller, John, 198
Wallian, Samuel Spencer, 187
Weatherston, Mary, 212
Weil, Simone, xi, 211
Welly (author's friend), 81, 86–87, 96
West Virginia, 105
Whole, 88
winter camper (self-amputation patient),
    56–60, 83

witchcraft, 201
Wolf, Mabel, 42–43
women, historical treatment of hysteria in,
    184–89, 190–93
Woolf, Virginia, 110–12
World War I, 184–85
Wrigley, Charles Harold, 1, 13, 16, 70
wrists, cutting of, 51–52

X-rays, 32

Yates, Andrea, 140–41, 143–45, 155,
    157, 158
Yates, Rusty, 157
youth, onset of mental illness in,
    76, 108

Christine Montross is an assistant professor of psychiatry and human behavior and the codirector of the Medical Humanities and Bioethics Scholarly Concentration at the Warren Alpert Medical School of Brown University. She is also a practicing inpatient psychiatrist. Montross's previous book, *Body of Work,* was named an Editors' Choice by the *New York Times* and one of the *Washington Post*'s best nonfiction books of 2007. She and her partner, the playwright Deborah Salem Smith, live in Rhode Island with their two young children.